ABOUT THE AUTHOR

Henrietta Branford's first Signature title, *The Fated Sky*, published to much accolade, was shortlisted for the Guardian Children's Fiction Award in 1997. She won the Smarties Prize for *Dimanche Diller* in 1994, also shortlisted for the Guardian Children's Fiction Award. She says: 'I started to write when I was forty and it's the best job I've ever tried. I live in Southampton, in the south of England, but I was born in India. My father was a soldier, and we soon moved to Jordan, where we lived in a house with a corrugated iron roof and a big hot garden. There were smooth cement floors and I used to lie on them to get cool, and paint pictures. Later we moved to the New Forest, which seemed dark and wet by comparison, but beautiful too.

'I went to lots of schools. I was not a good pupil. I've always read and imagined quite a lot, and my writing opens out of this.

'It takes a lot of people to make a book.'

Henrietta Branford

Chance of Safety

Henrietta Branford

Hodder
Children's
Books

a division of Hodder Headline plc

A Catalogue record for this book is available from the British Library

ISBN 0 340 69963 9

Typeset by Avon Dataset Ltd, Bidford-on-Avon, Warks

Printed and bound in Great Britain by
Clays Ltd, St Ives plc

Hodder Children's Books
A division of Hodder Headline plc
338 Euston Road
London NW1 3BH

One

The prisoner stooped lower, hunching her shoulders, trying to get away from the rain. Water bounced off the oily surface of the motorway, splashing her face and running down her neck. She worked as slowly as she could without attracting the attention of the foreman. She did not allow herself to think of tea or tobacco. You had to keep a steady rhythm. Make it look good. She sniffed, and wiped her nose on the sleeve of her jacket. Her head felt tight.

Each prisoner wore the latest in electronic tags: small hi-tech discs that contrasted oddly with the rags they wore – old coats, flapping overalls, strips of this or that wound round their heads to cover their cropped hair. They worked in silence. Men and women, black and white, all young; repaying their debt to society.

The prisoner sniffed again, and tasted blood. She thought about time – how fast it passes when times are good, how slowly when they're bad. She was fifteen and her last year had been her slowest. Fourteen was when she had decided to be pretty. Long hair. Gorgeous clothes – all nicked. Fourteen had gone by in about a fortnight. Seemed like she'd blinked and woken up in prison. She knew that sixteen wouldn't come.

A car slid past the prisoners, slowed by the road works, its warm interior bathed momentarily by the harsh white tower lights. The driver glanced at the line of prisoners and then looked away. The prisoners made her feel uncomfortable. Her son Alex, sitting beside her, caught the eye of a young woman – thin and white with a streak of red under her nose. Their eyes met and they stared at one another for a second. Then the car was gone, rain sluicing up from underneath its tyres, soaking the prisoner's legs.

'I wish they wouldn't make them work at night,' Ruth said. 'It's dangerous. You don't always see them in the dark.'

'It's their own fault. If they don't want to end up digging roads at midnight, they shouldn't nick and mug and deal and do the stuff they do.'

'I don't mind them being punished, Alex. I suppose society has to punish people who break the law. But is

2

this the way to do it? At night? In the rain?'

They drove on west, heading uphill. From where they lived, the town below looked pretty, especially at night. Tall blocks of flats rose like fairy towers out of dark, mysterious streets. You could not see, by night and from a distance, the boarded up windows, the blocked chutes, the rubbish piled in smelly heaps. On every stretch of open ground, where streets had been demolished, bonfires twinkled. Alex had heard there were huge groups of people – runners they were called – out there, living like savages. Thieves and murderers, people said. In summer, a blue haze of smoke hung over the whole east side of the city, where makeshift shacks straggled towards the airport. It looked busy, crowded, bustling. Alex supposed the people who lived down there must like it that way. Himself, he liked the space and style of his own wide, tree-lined street.

He followed his mother, Ruth, indoors just as his little sister Nelly came flying down the hall. Ludo, the family dog, plodded behind her, wearing a cowboy hat. Nelly's double holster and cap guns dangled round his neck and bumped against his broad and trusting chest. He looked resentful.

'Nelly! Take that stuff off Ludo,' Alex scolded. 'You know he hates being dressed up.'

'He doesn't mind. He likes it. He's being Deputy Dawg.'

Alex could never understand why Ludo put up with so much grief from Nelly. But then, most people did. He bent to rub behind the dog's ears. Nelly was six. Alex was ten years older. Ten good years, he thought. Then Nelly.

Most evenings, if Ruth was working late at the hospital, the family would eat out. Occasionally their father, Rob, would cook. Tonight was roast Welsh lamb cooked by Rob, with mint sauce made from fresh mint, redcurrant jelly, home-made gravy, roast potatoes and fresh green beans. Good food. Food for good times. But good times can change.

Anger blazing from the eyes of a dying prisoner changed Alex Kentigern's life. Well, that was part of it. But the death of one young prisoner lying alone on a high white bed would not in itself have been enough. What else?

The same month that Alex was to see the prisoner die, his father Rob, up in the executive suite of Motorways Incorporated, found a set of figures that did not add up. Rob pushed his glasses up his nose and clicked through the file on his screen. Somebody had been buying motorway materials on the cheap. Too cheap. Rob liked his figures to make sense. He trawled through several files on his computer. The stuff in question was mostly gravel for sub-base. Why was it cheap? Where had it come from? Rob would have no substandard materials used if he could help it. He began to make enquiries.

One corpse. A set of dodgy figures. What else? At work in her hospital, Ruth heard rumours of a new disease. No one seemed very interested. But then, no one who mattered seemed to be affected: the people who caught it – or did it catch them? – were all prisoners, young criminals working out their sentences on the roads. There were plenty more where they came from. But Ruth was interested. Ruth was interested in all forms of radiation and this disease looked to her like some new form of radiation sickness. Also, this form of radiation – if that was what it was – seemed to be following a particular stretch of motorway. Why?

Alex didn't know about the figures his father Rob had found. Or the research his mother Ruth had seen. Alex had worries of his own, to do with spots and money. How come he had so many of the first and hardly any of the second? A simple reversal of this state of affairs was all he wanted. Was that so much to ask? He was in his mother's office at the hospital, waiting for a lift home with her, the day the prisoner was brought in. A nurse put her head round the door.

'Hi, Alex. How's tricks? Doctor Ruth – I've got someone in isolation you might like to see. Looks like Road Sickness. Better go and see her now, she's further on than we expected. It's a nuisance, there won't be time for any of the tests you wanted done.' Alex tagged along behind his mother. He had never seen a really ill person.

The prisoner's face was emptied by disease. A smudge of red shadowed her upper lip like a child's milk moustache. Her body was a twist of bone wrapped in a waxy skin. An electronic tag shone on her skeletal wrist. She wanted to swear but she was long past swearing. *Mum*, she cried, silently. *Where are you? I want you, Mum.*

The look in the dying prisoner's eyes played a large part (given what an insubstantial thing a glance is) in getting Alex and his sister Nelly, Ruth, Rob, and Ludo into the family car a few months later, sleepy and grumpy in the early morning darkness. Heading away from home without a travel permit.

Two

The Police on Exit North didn't bother searching the car. They had just brewed the first cup of the day and they were not about to let it go cold. In any case, Rob's was a real Alpha Sector car – long and sleek and shiny. No need to search a car like that.

The sergeant stood stiff and respectful in his blue uniform – known to jokers as a fly suit, after the proverbial blue-arsed fly, because of the way the police were drawn to anything rotten and couldn't keep away from other peoples' business. The man checked Rob's local travel papers and glanced at his face. He checked again and called a colleague over. The colleague took Rob's papers and strolled over to his car. Next came the buzz and crackle of static.

Rob's hands were tense on the driving wheel. He began to swear, softly, under his breath. Ruth, sitting next to him, rested one hand on his knee, pressing gently: *Cool it.*

Rob's were city limit papers. They entitled him to drive within a ten mile radius of his home town. Everyone who drove a car had access to such papers. To go further, you bought an exit permit. Rob could have got one easily if he'd applied a month or two ago. But a month or two ago he hadn't known he'd want one. Papers are like that. By the time you know you want them it's too late to get them.

Everyone accepted that the rising tide of crime, together with the constant threat of terrorism, made tight travel regulation essential. Nobody wanted bands of thieves and beggars roaming the land. If your work required you to travel, you got an exit permit. If it didn't, you could always apply. Permits cost money, but Alpha Sector people had plenty of that. It was a small price to pay, if it helped fight crime.

The majority of the population were not, of course, affected one way or the other by travel restrictions or permits. Grunts don't travel.

What do you write on a Beta Sector School report?
Anything you like. The parents can't read.

What do you call a Beta Sector hospital?
A morgue.

Alex knew loads of grunt jokes. Nothing cruel. Just humour.

'Thank you, Sir.' The sergeant was smiling. So was Rob. It was done. They were through.

Alex looked back and saw the men silhouetted against their roadside fire. It was the sort men light in a bucket with holes in, and stand round, out of doors. One of the men was speaking into his radio, but Alex thought nothing of that.

They left the motorway nine miles north of where they'd joined it. 'It's going to be a long run,' Ruth warned. 'We'll take the back roads so we don't get asked to show our papers. And we won't be stopping much. Only when someone *has* to go, Nelly.'

'I don't want to go to Granny's house. She hasn't even got television. I hate Scotland. It always rains. *Why* do I have to go?'

'You know why, Nelly.'

Nelly sighed. She did. Her parents had explained everything. Boring.

Alex thought about the prisoner in the hospital. When she died, Ruth had put her arm round him and they had walked in silence back to her office. 'She was your age, Alex,' Ruth had said. 'Her skull hardly dented the pillow.'

What could anybody do, Alex had wondered, to make them deserve that? That wasn't punishment. That was murder. No, not murder. Accidental death. Because the authorities couldn't have known that she was going to catch Road Sickness. Could they?

The prisoner had been in reasonable health, for a Beta Sector Juvenile, when arrested. A bit overweight. Bad teeth. Poor muscle tone. Flat feet. Mildly anaemic. Nothing unusual. When she died, ten months later, she was suffering from vomiting and diarrhoea and her hair was falling out, though that was hard to tell with prisoners once their heads were shaved. Also she was bleeding from everywhere.

Rob, meanwhile, had found out why his sand and gravel was cut-price. It came from the site of a de-commissioned nuclear power plant and with it came toxic waste – chemicals and radioactive material. Left alone, the stuff was supposed to deteriorate gradually, becoming harmless at some unspecified point in the future – though Rob had his doubts about this. Dug up and sold to Motorways Incorporated for sub-base, it was unpredictable to say the least. Rob and Ruth put two and two together and came up with a thin girl dying on a high white bed.

Rob couldn't be the only one at work who knew about contaminated gravel. So: who else knew? Rob began to ask around to see who else had noticed. He did this carefully, asking a few good mates – people he felt inclined to trust. There had been a time, a long while back, when Rob would have contacted his MP. Or written to the papers. Or maybe, going back a little further, climbed up a tree or camped out in a tunnel. Now, there were no demonstrations. No MPs. No newspapers. No news.

Ruth shared Rob's information with a few good friends at the hospital. A pattern began to emerge. Then one evening, sorting out his desk, Rob found a note tucked inside some papers. *Take care*, it said. *They know you're interested.* There was no signature, only a drawing of a little dancing pin man. Rob had crossed the line that divided the law from the lawless. But he didn't know that yet.

The same week, someone came up to upgrade Ruth's computer. All of the department's computers were being upgraded, the engineer told her. She checked; hers was the only machine that was touched.

Next, Alex was accused of stealing CDs from his

college library. Two policemen came to search the house. 'Search where you like,' Ruth said. 'My son has never stolen anything in his life.'

The police went through the house taking books off shelves, lifting carpet, emptying drawers, unfolding sheets and towels from the bathroom cupboard, reading the messages on the pin board by the telephone, turning out Ruth's desk and Rob's shelf full of files. They even looked in Nelly's toy box. Alex wasn't worried, he knew he had nothing to hide.

Ruth made them tea and took it up to them – they were in Alex's room by then. They'd left it till last and they were making a meal of it. Piles of old socks and shirts, books, letters, boxes of diskettes from his home computer, were scattered on the floor. Ruth shook her head and left them to it. The room, she thought, looked not much worse than usual. When at last they came down to the kitchen, one of the policemen carried the teacups and the other held a stack of CDs. They said they'd found them wedged behind the headboard of Alex's bed. They said that Alex would be hearing from the courts.

'Did you steal those CDs, Alex?' Ruth asked.

Alex shook his head. He felt sick, bewildered.

'My son did not put those CDs there,' Ruth said, icily. 'If he says he didn't, he didn't. In which case someone else must have. I'll be lodging a complaint.'

'Lodge away, lady,' the policeman answered.

Ruth blushed red with anger. She was not used to being spoken to like that by anyone. Certainly not by a grunt.

'They put them there, Mum,' Alex said, when the police had gone. Ruth nodded. She was angry but she wasn't scared. Alex put his room back together and opened both the windows. Somehow, the place still felt dirty.

'Let's drive north and stay with Granny Kate in Scotland for a few days,' Rob suggested that evening. 'Would you like that, Alex?'

Alex was keen to go.

'What about permits?' Ruth asked. 'Permits will take for ever to come through.'

'Do they matter?' Alex asked.

'No permits, no petrol.'

'Dandy'll help us,' Rob said. 'Dandy can get his hands on anything. I think we should get away, just for a week.'

At the time, Alex didn't know about contaminated road materials, or the note Rob had found in his desk, or the research Ruth had seen, or the 'upgrading' of her computer at work. Also, he had not yet understood, and neither had his parents, that it was dangerous to be inquisitive. But his room felt dirty, and he liked visiting his grandmother in Scotland. And everybody knew that his uncle Dandy could fix anything. Dandy was Rob's older brother. He knew the right people. He had pull. He had a top job that carried every perk you could think of and several you couldn't. He had a big house. Best of all, he had Rachel, his clever, lovely wife.

Dandy had everything, until that spring, when Rachel took off, leaving nothing but a letter that he showed, weeping, to Rob and Ruth. *Sorry*, the letter said. *I'm off. I need fresh fields, and pastures new.* Rachel, it seemed, had a new man. It knocked the stuffing out of Dandy.

None of them could believe it. Ruth in particular found the letter strange. 'Rachel was such a scholar,' she told Rob. 'She loved Milton. She would have laughed at me if I'd misquoted him like that.'

Rob looked confused.

'Fresh *woods*, Rob, not fresh fields. *Tomorrow to fresh*

woods, and pastures new. Rachel would know that, Rob.'

'Why would she worry about Milton?' Rob replied. 'She was walking out on Dandy. Leaving him to join her new lover, by the sound of it. She had more on her mind than Milton.'

'It just doesn't seem like her. None of it does.'

Three

Dandy brought petrol, plenty of it. And a load of firewood to hide in the trailer full of supplies they were taking up to Kate Kentigern. He said it was easy to get off the exit roads without a permit – he'd done it lots of times.

'Go on, Rob,' he advised. 'Take a break. Let the dust settle down here. Go and see Mum for a few days – it's time one of us did. And on the way, why don't you check out that stretch of road where your sub-base has gone? You'll be going right past it. Keep me in touch, Rob. Let me know if you find anything interesting. I care too, you know.'

Dandy had looked more wretched than ever. 'Come too,' Ruth begged. 'You need to get away as much as we do. More. And Kate would love to have you both under her roof.' But Dandy wouldn't.

Once the Check Point on Exit North was passed,

Alex and Nelly slept until Ruth leaned back and shook them gently awake.

'Sorry,' she said. 'I know it was an early start. But there are some things that we have to talk about.' Alex stretched within the confines of his seat belt. Nelly wiped dribble from her chin and rubbed her eyes. 'I want to tell you what I'm going to say if anybody asks us where we're going. Or if anybody comes to Granny Kate's house and asks why we're there. Police or anyone else. OK? Nelly – are you listening? Because I'm not going to talk about the police coming to our house. Or anything that Dad and I found out.' Alex prodded his sister awake again. 'I'm going to say that Gran's not well, and we're going to take care of her for a while until she's better. And if anybody happens to ask you, you say that too. OK, Alex? Nelly?'

'Is Granny Kate ill?' Nelly asked. 'Why didn't you tell me before? I would have done her a picture.'

'She isn't ill. She's fine. But just so we have a good reason to be visiting, in case anyone asks, we're going to *say* she's ill.'

Nelly said nothing. She was intrigued by the idea of being told by her mother to lie. She rather liked it, on the whole, but it left her a little confused. Alex was

17

more pragmatic. 'What do we say is wrong with Gran?' he asked.

'Back trouble,' Ruth said. 'Which is true in a way. She often does have back trouble.'

Rob took his eyes off the road briefly and glanced over his shoulder. 'So, Nelly,' he said. 'If people stopped the car right now and asked you why you weren't at school, what would you say?'

'Mind your own business?'

'Come on, Nell. It's important.'

'I'd say my Granny has a bad back. She can't get the coal in for her fire and stuff. So we're staying with her until she's better. Because Mum's a doctor.'

'Nice touch about the coal,' Rob said. 'Well done.'

Rob pulled over at midday for a lunch break and they ate sandwiches sitting in a row with their backs to a stone wall, looking out across a valley. Afterwards, Ruth drove and Rob read the map. 'We're eight kilometres from where my sub-base went to,' he said. 'Take the next turning left.'

'I don't want to go back on the motorway,' Ruth said. 'It's asking for trouble.'

'It's crazy not to take a look.'

The prisoners were half way through a twelve hour shift. Most were experienced hands, working slowly, reserving their energy. Newcomers who worked fast to impress the foreman would not be on their feet come midnight.

Two identical shrimps, working side-by-side at the back of the line, were closest to the car when Ruth pulled off between the traffic cones and parked. They were taking ant-sized bites out of a mountain of gravel. Neither one looked up when Rob got out and walked towards the foreman, but Alex saw them watching, sideways, their stringy arms still shovelling. Their faces were splattered with watery red gravel dust and sweat had cleared runnels down their faces, making dirty marmalade stripes. One of them caught Alex's eye and looked away. Both had prison haircuts. Both wore reddish-brown rags. Both had dried grass stuffed into their boots instead of socks. They didn't look much older than Nelly. They worked in a synchronised choreography of boredom – hunch and swing, sniff, sleeve under nose, hunch and swing, shuffle, sniff.

The foreman's mobile home was parked down in the corner of a muddy field with two long, squat prisoners' sheds behind it. A dismal fire smoked on a hearth made out of breeze blocks and a huge man sat beside it on a broken chair. He looked at home, sitting outdoors by a stretch of muddy motorway, poking a fire with a stick. His long hair was tied back in a ponytail and he wore mud-coloured overalls unzipped down the front to allow his mighty belly to flow outwards between massive knees. The backs of his hands were covered with tattoos, writhing in a blue stream up his forearms to disappear under his rolled-up sleeves. Alex and Rob walked over to the fire. The foreman looked up, then leaned forward and poked the fire.

Rob said hello, and the man grunted. 'I work for the firm that's resurfacing this stretch of road,' Rob began.

'That's funny,' the foreman said, 'I thought my young prisoners was doing that.'

'I guess they are. But we supply the materials.' Rob held out a business card.

'No good to me, mate. I can't read.'

'I want to take some samples,' Rob went on. 'Gravel. Sand. A bit of black top.'

'Help yourself, mate.'

Rob nodded. 'Something's making these prisoners sick,' he said. 'And I want to know what it is. My wife's a doctor. She wants to know too.'

The foreman nodded and spat into the fire. 'You, me an' her,' he said. 'They're all bleedin'. You can't see it cause of the red earth, but they are. I shall be too, before long. You reckon sommat in the sand of the gravel's makin' 'em sick?'

'I didn't say that. This is not an official enquiry. It's just a personal interest, really.'

The foreman looked Rob in the eye and laughed. It was an extraordinarily frank and open sound, as though he felt entitled to do and say exactly what he chose. There was no fear in it. It was a long time since Rob had heard anybody laugh like that and he found himself smiling right back into the man's eyes.

'Don't fret,' the man said. 'Don't tell my boss and I won't tell yours.' He took a tin of tobacco from his overall pocket and rolled two thin tailor-mades, leaned back on his broken chair and held one out to Rob. On the back of his left hand, a little blue pin-man tattoo danced. The same little pin man who'd been dancing at the bottom of that note on Rob's desk.

'I don't smoke. But thank you,' Rob said, staring at the tattoo.

'Wise man. No need to make yourself sick is there? Plenty out there willin' to do it for you.' He lit up and inhaled. 'You got a personal interest in prisoners, 'ave you?' he asked.

'No. But I feel responsible in a way. I work for the firm that supplies the materials.'

'Well, I'll tell you this. They're all right when they get 'ere. They're all right for a month or two. Then they get sick. All of 'em do, sooner or later. Sometimes the sickest of 'em gets away from 'ere to somewhere a bit more comfortable. I do what I can. But it don't do no good. They all die in the end.'

'What do you think is happening?'

'I don't think nothin'. I don't know. I'm an ignorant man. You take your samples, you're the big boss. Do it now, while nobody's about.'

Rob fetched a trowel and a set of tin boxes with lids. He took a trowel full of each of the materials on site while Alex held the boxes. Both of them were careful not to get mud on their hands. Two police cars cruised by slowly, antennae waving, just as they were finishing. They slowed to scan the prisoners but showed no interest in Rob or Alex. Neither did they acknowledge an ironic salute from the foreman, slouching beside his fire.

Back in the car, Ruth shook with anger and fear. 'I knew we shouldn't have done this. What if they'd stopped and asked to see our papers?'

Rob put his arm round her shoulders. 'They didn't. We're fine. It's OK, Ruth.'

After that, Alex listened to music on his personal stereo and slept. When he woke it was evening and they were passing through a small grey town that looked familiar. His grandmother's house, hot food, warm beds, were only forty kilometres away. Meanwhile the rain slashed down turning the tarmac oily black. Ruth made a sharp left turn, opposite the library, and drove down the tiny, winding lane. She changed down and slowed the car to a crawl, cornering carefully because of the wet road, pulled gently round a bend and found herself confronting half a dozen men strung out across the road. An assortment of nasty-looking dogs leaned on taut leather leashes. Two people, roped together, stumbled along the verge. When one of them staggered and swayed too far off vertical, the other straightened him up with a gentle shove. Somewhere a radio crackled.

'Don't stop!' Rob hissed. 'Drive on through them!'

'I can't! I'll hit someone!'

'Do it!'

Something heavy hit the radiator and Ruth slowed

to a standstill. Rob reached across to flick the central locking on. Alex released his and Nelly's seat belts. Nelly shut her eyes and pushed her face hard into Alex's shoulder. The car rocked as the lock on Ruth's door smashed and a man leaned in and yanked her out onto the road. Ludo exploded in the back and Nelly screamed. Ruth was shoved down onto the slippery road and the man stood over her, one heavy boot next to her hand on the wet tarmac. Rob leapt to reach her and was knocked off balance by a blow to his head. He went down beside her on the wet pavement, heavy boots thudding into him. His hands were yanked behind his back and handcuffs fastened on his wrists. Ruth's mouth was open in a shout of rage and fear, her face was wet with tears and rain, her hair stuck to her head. Nelly stared, horrified, shouting at Alex to make it all stop. Alex was frozen, helpless, in the back of the car. He knew he should get out and stand beside his parents. Just to be there. Just to be with them. But he couldn't make himself do it.

A man pushed head and shoulders into the car, stinking it out with dirt and tobacco. 'You! Out!' he grunted, hauling Alex out by the jacket.

'Alex!' Nelly wailed. 'Wait!'

The man reached back and slapped her. 'You too!

Quick! And shut it!' He hauled her out, cuffing Ludo back. Round at the trailer somebody was lifting out Rob's samples.

Rob's eyes were fixed on Ruth's face, questioning. Ruth nodded. Both of them looked across at Alex. Ruth mouthed *run*. Alex blinked. Run where? A flock of Nelly's paper dolls blew past. Alex kept his eyes on Rob's face, begging for answers. Rob's eyes flicked over the hedge and away. He lifted his chin a fraction and whistled. Ludo shot from the back of the car all teeth and bristles, growling insults at the other dogs. Men waded in cuffing and shouting and Ludo went down snarling. The gap in the men's attention was big enough, for a few seconds, to let Alex go.

Somehow he found the strength to run. He grabbed his sister by the hand and leapt, towing Nelly behind him, over the ditch, through the hedge and away. He ran without thinking or looking back, leaving the sound of the dog fight behind, past the low white church and through the graveyard, up and over the slippery ridges of a wide ploughed field, towing Nelly behind him, away from the road and the town and the men, away from his father's bruised face and his mother's white hand on the wet black road.

When the field ended and trees rose dark ahead, he

dived under them, pulling Nelly with him. For a while they lay panting and crying under the dripping leaves. 'Alex? Why did those men hit Dad?' Nelly asked, when she could speak.

'I don't know, Nell.'

'You should have helped them, Alex.'

'How?'

'You shouldn't have run away.'

Alex felt guilt and weakness wash over him. He should have stayed, not run. But Ruth said *run*. Rob meant him to as well. Both of them wanted him to take Nelly and run. If he had stayed, they'd all be prisoners now. Fury replaced his guilt. 'Oh yea? If they'd got me as well, what would you have done? I'd like to see you cope alone!' He gave Nelly a shove with all his pent-up misery behind it. She tipped over backwards on the wet earth and they both cried, leaning away from one another, alone with their fear. Alex stopped first. He held fast in his mind's eye to the image of his parents. He could see them clearly, but already they were a tiny bit further off.

'Don't cry, Nelly,' he said, after a while. 'It won't help. They'll be OK. One phone call to Dandy and it'll all be sorted out. We'll be fine too. I promise you.'

'What are we going to do?'

'We'll go to Gran's house. Mum and Dad will come and find us there.'

'I want Mum, not you, Alex. Let's go back and make them let her go.'

'Don't be stupid, Nell. How can we do that?'

'You tell me if you're so clever! You're not in charge of me! I want Mum and Dad, I don't want you!'

'I suppose you can find your way to Gartbeg by yourself, can you?'

'I'm not going to Granny's house.'

'Yes you are. And I know the way. You don't.'

'Bet you don't either, big head.'

'I do. We can hitch.'

'We're not allowed. *You're* not even allowed. What if those people see us?'

'They won't if we stay off the roads.'

'You said we could hitch.'

Nelly was still hiccuping and shaking. Alex rocked her, pushing down his own fear as best he could. Then he heard breathing, close by. Soft and steady. He nearly died until he realised it was Nelly. There was no orange glow of street lights on the clouds to light the night. Just darkness and rain. In the end he slept too. He dreamed that something big was following him. He

could hear it, coming along behind him, slow and sure.
But he couldn't see what it was.

Four

Alex woke with a shock to find daylight shining through the branches. He'd slept all night. Fear flooded back, along with misery. Ruth, mouth open, crying. Rob, hunched down under a rain of kicks. How could he have slept? Anything could have happened, and all he'd done was sleep. He crawled out of the hollow and stood staring back across the brown furrowed field. He was bursting for a pee.

'Alex! Wait for me!' Nelly had woken too. 'Alex, I'm hungry.'

'I've got a Mars Bar. D'you want half?' When did Nelly ever not want half a Mars Bar?

'Don't go without me, Alex. I'm coming too.'

'I'm only going for a pee.'

'I need one too.'

'Find your own place. I don't want you going right beside me.'

'I'm scared on my own. I can't go if I'm scared. And there isn't any paper.'

'Use leaves.'

Nelly began to cry. Alex looked at her and sighed. She looked so small. How was he ever going to get her to their grandmother's? 'It's OK, Nelly. You can come with me.'

Stumbling through the early morning wood with Nelly clutching his hand and rain still dripping off the trees all round them, Alex realised that he was going to have to keep his own fear hidden. He must somehow keep it wrapped up inside himself, where Nelly couldn't feel it, if he was going to keep her calm, keep both of them moving forward. *I can do that*, he told himself. But for how long?

They left the wood with the grey church spire behind them in the east and travelled zigzag over open fields, keeping close in to ditches and hedges, ready to dive for shelter. Each time they found a stream, Alex made Nelly hold hands and walk in it beside him until their feet were rubbed sore on their shoes and their legs were frozen. Nelly cried and moaned, but Alex would not let her off. 'Do it, Nell. It's to keep us safe. It'll put those people's dogs off our scent, so they can't follow us.'

'Are their dogs chasing us, Alex?'

'I don't know. They might be. But they won't catch us, Nelly, if we do this.'

Both of them were soon exhausted, more from fear than from walking. Round about dinner time they stopped in a field of carrots. Alex pulled some up and washed them in the ditch.

'I don't want them raw,' Nelly complained. 'I like them cooked, with salt and butter.'

Alex snapped. 'Eat them or don't eat,' he said. 'I don't care which.'

'Will we be at Granny's tonight, Alex? Will we have supper at Granny's?'

'No.'

'Where are we going to sleep?'

'I'll find us somewhere. We'll be all right, Nelly. I can take care of us.'

Nelly was silent. Her hair stuck out round her ears and her bottom lip began to wobble. Alex put his arm round her and rested his chin on her head. She shook him off and ate her carrots, putting one in her pocket for later. Then they went on, heading towards the line of hills that lay between them and safety.

Late that afternoon they smelled smoke and Nelly

persuaded Alex to let them take a look; they crept along, keeping well down behind a hedge. Presently they saw a wild-haired woman with two small children, all three of them very dirty. The woman had pitched a little tent down in the corner of a field and she was cooking something. The children were playing 'scissors, paper, stone'. Both of them screamed with laughter every time they won. The woman watched them while she cooked, smiling each time they laughed. Alex thought he and Nelly were well hidden, but she soon looked up and called to them.

'You can come out from behind that hedge you know. I won't eat you.'

The children stopped their game and stared. 'We eat rabbits,' one said.

'And potatoes.'

'And biscuits when Mumma can nick 'em.'

'But we don't eat people 'cos we're not Hannibal cannibals!'

They lay on their backs with their feet in the air and laughed.

'All we've had today,' Nelly said angrily, 'is raw carrots.'

'Is that so, pet? Where are you going to?'

'We're going to Gartbeg. To our grandmother's,' Alex replied.

'Because she's ill. With a bad back,' Nelly put in. 'She can't get out to fetch her coal in.'

'You on your own?'

Alex nodded.

'We were with Mum and Dad,' Nelly added. 'But some men pulled them out of the car and Dad told Alex to run away. With me.'

Alex frowned at her. Why must she tell everybody everything?

'Was it bluebottles did that?' the woman asked. Her children ran round in small circles buzzing.

'I don't know. I think so,' Alex replied.

The woman eased a piece of wood in under the pot on the fire. 'Don't fret,' she said, tugging a wisp of Nelly's hair. 'If it was bluebottles, they're bound to let your mam and daddy go. They don't want posh folk cluttering up the cells.'

The woman gave them hot food – it was stew. She had one tin plate, which Nell and Alex shared while she and her children ate from the pot. 'Pigeon, that is,' she said.

'How d'you catch them?' Nell asked, running her finger round the rim of the plate.

'Shoot 'em,' the woman said. Nelly looked impressed.

'Can we stay with you for tonight?' she asked.

'*Nelly* . . .' Alex hissed. But the woman nodded.

'You're welcome to a bit of our fire.'

'I've seen people like you,' Nelly announced. 'On telly. You're a beggar.'

'I am,' the woman laughed. 'But I don't think it's me doing the begging just now.'

'Why don't you live in a house?' Nelly asked. 'Like proper people do?'

'Couldn't pay the rent. Stinking hole it was anyway – didn't fancy staying, did we kids? We stay here and there now. We stay with the runners.'

'What runners?'

'You'll find out,' the woman said. She'd say no more than that. Runners were not people you talked about to anyone who didn't know them. Not even lost bedraggled kids like these. If you wanted the runners to help you, you helped the runners. By keeping quiet about who they were – and where they were.

The children were sucking condensed milk out of a tin. They gave Nelly a suck, and she handed the tin to Alex. Later, Alex and Nelly slept by her fire, rolled into a warm dirty rug the woman lent them. In the morning she gave them hot tea with no milk and cold baked potatoes. 'Get back onto the road, so you don't get lost,' she said. 'Cross-country's harder, you'll not manage that. But hop off through the hedge each time you hear a car coming, just in case the bluebottles are looking for you. Good luck.'

They said goodbye and the woman packed up her belongings and went off across the fields, the children trotting behind like small, neat animals.

By midday Alex and Nelly were back on the right road. They had only dived through the hedge once, and that was for an old farm van with a sheep dog lolling out of the back. Nelly made less fuss than Alex had expected. When they came to a cottage with an apple tree in the front garden, Nelly wanted to knock on the door and ask for some fruit but Alex wouldn't have that.

'No way,' he said. 'You don't know who the people are. I'm going to climb the tree and get as many apples as I can. You stay here. Shout to me if you see anybody coming, and run. Don't wait for me to get down out of the tree. Just run. OK?'

'That's stealing, Alex. And the people will be cross. Anyway I don't want apples. I want egg and chips.'

'Shut up and let me get some apples.'

The tree was halfway between the house and the road, standing between neat beds of flowers and vegetables on either side of a path. Alex was up, pockets bulging, when Nelly shouted. He took his eyes off the branch he was clinging to and saw a tall old woman watching him from the open front door. One gnarly hand shaded her eyes as she peered up into the tree. Alex jumped, the front of his jacket knobbly and stuffed with her apples. He felt embarrassed and ashamed but not afraid. The woman was old, and looked slow on her feet. Nelly meanwhile remembered that she was supposed to run, turned, caught her foot on something and went flying. She sat for a second with her mouth open, rubbing her knees. Then she began to holler.

The old woman shook her head and started towards Nelly. 'Come here then,' she said. 'Show me that knee. Come on. I won't hurt you.' Nelly hobbled over to her. So much for being careful, Alex thought. The woman bent down slowly to examine the knee saying 'there there' and 'never mind'. There wasn't a mark on it but she smiled at Nelly and patted her cheek. Nelly smiled back. 'Hungry, are you?' the old woman asked. 'Best come indoors if you are.'

Alex pushed thoughts of Hansel, Gretel and the witch in the gingerbread house firmly out of his head and followed Nell inside. The house smelled dusty and quiet, of polish and wood fires and long lives. In the small front room old photos, framed in heavy wooden frames, hung on the walls revealing old, blurred people from long ago. Pink Albertine roses, cut from the garden, dropped petals from a vase. A clock ticked. In front of the hearth a sleeping cat twitched one ear towards the door.

'I'm sorry about the apples,' Alex said.

'That's all right, my duck,' the woman said. 'You're not the first hungry lad to pinch a few apples. Nor the last.' Her round glasses were mended with pink elastoplast and her hair was jammed back behind two hair grips. She wore slippers that fastened with Velcro and a faded overall. Alex let go of Nelly's hand and began to fish apples from his pockets, putting them down on the sideboard. The old woman watched, smiling and shaking her head. Alex realised that he felt safe, in her house.

'I'm sorry,' he said again. 'For trying to take your apples.'

'Is it the first time you've been hungry?' the old woman asked.

'Yes,' Alex answered, with surprise. '*This* hungry, anyway.'

'Well, hunger's a hard master. It'll make you do all manner of things you wouldn't do without it. Taking apples from a tree's the least of them.'

When she made tea with milk and sugar and cut slices of bread and butter, Alex found it hard not to put his head down and guzzle off the plate. Nelly didn't even try not to. The old woman's name was Mary. She said her husband's name was Donald, but that he was away with his lorry and wouldn't be back till late. She had a Scots accent, but not the same as Kate Kentigern's. She cooked egg and chips and Alex refused to catch Nelly's eye. Mary watched them with pleasure.

'Where are you headed now?' she asked, when they had finished eating.

'We're going north. To Gartbeg,' Alex told her.

'To stay with our granny,' Nelly added.

'That's nice for your granny, my duck,' Mary said. 'And you're in luck, too, because my Donald's got a load of sheep to take over that way, tomorrow or the next day. You can go with him if you like. You'll be safer that way.'

Food, Alex thought. *Shelter. Transport. This time tomorrow we'll be there.*

He and Nelly climbed into an old saggy bed in the back bedroom that night. Downstairs, the door banged, and Donald came in. A chair scraped as he sat to eat. Afterwards, their two old voices flowed quietly on. 'So many bairns on the road,' Alex heard Mary say. 'Poor mites. They're old before their time, worn out with fear and hunger.'

'It's bad times we live in,' Donald answered. 'But we'll see better too, before we're gone.'

'D'you think so, Donald?'

'I do.'

Nelly cried and couldn't stop. Long after she had cried herself to sleep, Alex lay awake, thinking about his mother down on the road with the man's boot by her hand. And his father getting a kicking. He wondered what made Donald think that anything would change.

In the morning when Alex and Nelly went downstairs, Donald was sitting at the table eating toast and honey. He wore an ancient, felted-up blue jersey that made his red face look redder and his white hair whiter. Nell went straight over and sat down without being asked.

'Morning, ma'am,' the old man said, passing her a

slice. 'Come on,' he said, nodding to Alex. 'You too.'

Alex sat down, meaning to eat only a little, but the whole loaf was gone and the honey was halfway down the jar by the time he and Nelly had finished. Donald didn't seem to mind.

'Mary says you're going to your grandma's,' he said presently. 'No doubt she's worrying about you. Grandmas do.' He winked at Mary. 'Any road, I'm going over that way myself this morning. Got a load of sheep to pick up. Take 'em over towards Gartbeg once the paperwork's done. Permits for sheep you need now. It'll be permits for fleas next. I'll take you with me if you like.'

'That would be great,' Alex replied. 'You've been very kind to us. I don't know how to thank you. I haven't got any money . . .'

Donald laughed, and Alex blushed. First he came here stealing apples. Now he was saying that he'd pay them, if he could, for what they'd given freely, because they were that sort of people.

Nelly looked up, unconcerned. 'They don't mind, Alex,' she said. 'They don't mind whether we've got any money or not. They like helping people.'

'Little maid's right,' Donald observed.

Only as they were saying goodbye to Mary at the door did Alex notice, tiny on the doorstep, a little dancing pin man scratched into the stone.

'You've seen the dancing man,' Mary observed. 'Do you know what he means?'

Alex shook his head.

'Where you see him you'll find help. Best not to ask questions – but where you see him, you'll rest safe among friends.'

Alex shook hands, not knowing what else to do, but Mary leaned over and kissed him on the cheek, her skin paper-dry against his, a faint smell of soap rising from her faded overall.

The journey with Donald was slow and noisy. The cab filled with the smell of hot oil, the engine groaned up every hill, the windscreen wipers swished, and Nelly snored. Donald said little. Once they passed two gaunt dogs trotting one behind the other on the road and he turned to Alex and shook his head.

'Take care when you see dogs like that,' he said.

'I don't mind dogs,' Alex replied.

'I like them,' Nelly added. 'Dogs are better than people.'

'A dog can be your friend,' Donald agreed. 'And a good one, too. But when they're hungry, just like us, they behave differently. They go wild, and pack together, and then you must watch out for them. Those two have killed any number of sheep and cattle round here. And they'd kill more than sheep and cattle too, if they got the chance.'

Five miles out of Stepgavie, they turned off the road and drove down a muddy farm track. 'This is where I get the sheep from,' Donald said. 'Pick 'em up here, take 'em to town, get their papers sorted and take 'em on to a farm over by Gartbeg. You two may as well stay dry while we load up.'

The sheep were penned in a yard at the end of the track, in front of a low, dilapidated farm house. Their broad backs were beaded with rain. A woman wearing a heavy tweed coat and a man's peaked cap leaned on a stick, two dogs at her feet. Donald dropped the ramp at the back of the lorry, the woman whistled to her dogs, opened the yard gate, and in a matter of minutes the sheep were loaded.

Nelly watched it all. 'Ludo couldn't do that,' she told Donald as they set off again. 'He's our dog. He's with Mum and Dad.' She put her head down in Alex's lap and lay, thumb to mouth, eyes open, looking miserable. Donald fished in his jacket pocket and passed her a peppermint.

'Taste as good as your thumb that will,' he said.

Nelly unwrapped it, bit it in half and gave half to Alex. The old man nodded approvingly. 'Good lass,' he said. 'Share and share alike.' Nelly shut her eyes and sucked.

Five

Alex woke up suddenly when Donald turned off the engine. He saw that they were parked outside what looked like council offices in a little market town.

'We're at Stepgavie,' Donald told him. 'Stop in the cab while I'm inside. I'll be a wee while, but we'll have something to eat when the paperwork's done.'

Nelly was still asleep, dribbling peppermint spit onto Alex's leg. She didn't wake up until Donald came back a good hour later with two official-looking men behind him. 'They've come to count the sheep,' he told her. 'Got trouble sleeping, see. Not like you.' Nelly smiled. One of the men went round to the back of the lorry and began to peer in through the slats. The other walked up to the cab and opened the door.

'Get down, you two,' he said. Donald frowned. Alex and Nelly didn't move. 'Now. Not tomorrow. You'll need to come inside and get your travel permits stamped.'

'They've got no permits,' Donald said. 'They're only along for the ride.'

'Family, are they?'

Donald nodded.

The man leaned in and spoke past Alex to Nelly. 'What's your name, love?'

'Nelly Kentigern,' Nelly said, her accent sounding posh and strange and southern.

'Well, Nelly Kentigern. You and your brother better come with me. Your mum and dad are looking for you.'

Nelly slid down out of the cab, her face glowing. Alex jumped down and stood beside her, ready to grab her and run. On the surface, there was no obvious danger: A small-time official in a little market town, asking to see their travel permits. From what Donald had said there were dozens of scruffy kids on the road. What difference could two more make to this man? And yet, Alex sensed danger.

'Got the Kentigern kids here,' the man called to his mate behind the lorry. A radio crackled, then everything was quiet except for the sheep. The bleating stopped for a few seconds and Alex heard a voice distorted by the radio say: 'Hold them.'

Donald heard it too. 'Is that man of yours fiddling with my doors at the back?' he asked quickly. 'Only they're temperamental. Fly open at a touch, they do.' He hurried round the back of the lorry and kicked one of the doors. It dropped straight down onto the road, forming a ramp and out poured about fifty pent-up sheep. 'Damn and blast your man!' he swore. 'Will you look what he's done now!' The sheep had spread out and were milling round the little square. 'Fine sheep, Herdwick,' Donald added, thoughtfully. 'But not biddable.'

The man with the radio lunged at Nelly. Alex yanked her back out of his reach and ran – straight through the plunging, baa-ing flock and out the other side. Voices shouted after him – Donald's deep bellow: '*Run laddie, run!*' The other man's angry '*Get back here!*' Alex dragged Nell down the first side street he saw and they belted along, turning left and right, not daring to slow down. He didn't let her stop or slow until he was certain nobody was following. They were out of the middle of the town by then and running on windy, rubbish-strewn grass with tall blocks of flats ahead of them. Nelly was crying hard, still half believing Ruth and Rob were back there, waiting for her.

A group of boys standing around a pile of burning tyres looked up and shouted something. Alex caught Nelly's hand again and yanked her back into a run but two of the boys were up and after him. One grabbed him from behind and pulled him down onto the ground. Nelly slipped, screamed, and went over in the mud as she tried to dodge the other. The rest came up and stood round, spitting and staring, waiting for the lad who had caught Alex to make a move. Alex kept still, the boy's knee pressing into his back. Nelly was crying now. If it was money they wanted, they were going to be angry when they found out he had none. What would they do? Give him a beating probably. Alex had never had a beating. And Nelly? Surely they wouldn't touch Nelly? Before Alex could think any worse thoughts, a woman came out from the bottom of a block of flats.

'Leave those kids alone!' she hollered. 'Now! Or I'll let the caretaker's dog out after you!'

'Mates of yours, are they?' one of the boys called back.

'She 'asn't got any mates,' another said. 'Only in the jungle.'

But they moved back a little all the same. They began a jumping, grunting dance round Alex and Nelly, swinging their arms and making monkey noises. Either the woman shouting, or the threat of the caretaker's dog, had punctured the boys' aggression. Alex felt the knee lift off his back and stood up. The boys' circle widened until they were no longer standing round two prisoners; they were just fooling around.

The woman came over. She wore a woolly hat and an old coat half buttoned up around the baby she was carrying. One fat brown cheek and some soft black lambswool hair were all that showed.

'You don't want to hang round with this bunch of morons,' she advised, scooping Nelly to her feet. The ring of youths drifted away, still grunting and messing around, but no longer threatening. 'You'd best bring that littl'un indoors to my place to get her breath back,' she added to Alex. 'I live on the ninth floor. I came down to fetch water. You can help me carry it back up.'

Two plastic containers stood beside a standpipe over by the entrance to the flats. Alex took one and the young woman took the other. Together they struggled up nine flights of smelly concrete stairs; the woman fished a bunch of keys out of her pocket and undid the three locks on her boarded-up door. Inside the place was dark and smelly. All the windows were smashed.

An old wood-burning stove stood beside one of them, with a pipe sticking out through a sheet of tin that covered where the glass had been. A couple of broken car seats and a mattress sagged beside it. When the woman took off her coat and dropped it, Alex expected it to stand up on its own, it was so stiff with dirt, but instead it keeled over sideways and collapsed. She lifted her baby out of her sling and sank onto a car seat. Then she pulled off her hat, revealing brown and green and yellow plaits.

'You're not from round here, are you?' she asked, untangling coat and mittens from the baby. Alex shook his head. 'Sit down. Catch your breath. Don't let those apes out there upset you.'

Alex and Nelly sat side by side on the old car seats. Nelly's knees were wet with mud, her face was streaked and blotchy. Alex put his arm round her and hugged her gently. 'It's OK, Nell,' he said. He told the young woman only that they had been on their way to their grandmother's house.

'Where does she live?' the woman asked.

'Gartbeg,' Nelly told her. 'That's in Scotland.'

'You're in Scotland now, pet. But Gartbeg's a few miles from here. How are you going to get there?' she asked.

'We can walk,' Alex replied.

'I can't,' Nelly said.

The woman laughed. 'Well you haven't got to start out right now, pet. You stay the night, rest up a bit, and I'll find you some food before you go on. My name's Maggie. What's yours?'

'Nelly. And my brother's Alex.'

'Is that your baby?' Nelly asked. 'Is it a girl? What's her name?'

'Her name's Dayo. It means *joy arrives*, in her dad's language. He called her that. She's a joy to me all right, but her dad's gone.'

Maggie lit a fire in the wood burner – she had a stack of old pallets beside it which she smashed up with a hatchet till they were small enough to fit through the door of the stove.

'Got any food yourselves?' she asked.

Alex shook his head.

'I have,' Nelly said. She held out Donald's sandwiches. 'I didn't steal them. I was just holding them when that man pulled us out of the lorry. Mum and Dad weren't there, were they, Alex?'

'No. He was trying to trick us.' Alex explained, briefly, what had happened.

'Never trust a bluebottle, my pet,' Maggie advised.

'Now. Food. I've got two onions, four carrots, a spud and some dried peas. You've got sandwiches. We'll have soup and sandwiches. Nelly – can you take Dayo for me?'

Nelly sat on the mattress with Dayo on her lap while Alex and Maggie peeled and chopped for the soup. 'She's nice,' Nelly said, rubbing her tearstained cheek against Dayo's silky hair.

Once the soup was simmering on top of the stove, Alex helped Maggie get the place ready for the night. They pulled three bolts across the door and pushed a heavy chest of drawers against it. Maggie adjusted the sheets of tin round the stove pipe where it poked out the window and made sure the other windows were covered properly. Then she took a piece of cloth and spread it over a wooden pallet on the floor. She lit a candle and put it in a saucer in the middle.

'Right,' she said. 'Let's eat.'

'Can I give Dayo a bit of sandwich?' Nelly asked.

'Try her on a wee scrap,' Maggie said. Dayo took it, gummed it and spat it out. Her soft cheeks gleamed in the candlelight.

'Have a drop more, my love,' her mother coaxed taking her baby from Nelly. 'One for your Mammy and one for your Daddy and none for the bad men who took him away.'

51

'Where is her father?' Alex asked. 'Who took him away?'

'Police. They took all the foreign students. I tried everything to hide Moyo – but how do you hide a black man in a white town? I was so scared they'd find him. I made him stay indoors day and night, told everybody he'd left me, run off, and I didn't know where he was. I smuggled his food in as best I could. It was bad for him, waiting here all day, with me lugging Dayo up and down the stairs, looking for food. Moyo felt bad all the time because he couldn't help us, he couldn't even help himself. It was a dreadful time for us, the worst. We fought, shouted at one another, cried. What wouldn't I give now, to have him back to shout at just once? If a few more people had been on our side we might have made it. Some folk helped us. But most of them didn't bother. Some were too scared, I guess. Some hate foreigners. In the end one of them must have told on us.'

Maggie stopped talking and hugged Dayo tightly for a while. 'They came banging into my place. Kicked the door down. Dayo was screaming. So was I. They pulled Moyo out from behind the wardrobe and threw him on the floor. Knelt on his chest, half strangled him. I thought they were going to kill him. They hit him, and handcuffed him, and dragged him down the stairs. He was looking back up at us, shouting something I couldn't understand. They hit him again and he must have passed out. I don't even know what he was trying to say to us.'

The room was quiet for a while. Dayo whimpered. 'Where did they take him?' Alex asked.

'To the old fish canning place. I went there. It was full of foreigners. The last I saw of Moyo was his face looking at me from the back of the coach. He was all swollen up round the eyes. But he smiled at us. Blew Dayo a kiss. I thought it was the end of the world. But I had a child to care for. And I've managed.'

Alex looked round at the bare, crusty floors, the stained mattress, the boarded-up windows, the barricaded door. Maggie was proud of this. She was managing.

'I've tried to keep my head down, in case they come for Dayo. She's the wrong colour and folk know we're here. I know I've got to move, sooner or later.'

'Where will you go?'

'Maybe I'll join the runners.'

'I've heard about them. Who are they? What are they like?'

'You'll see, if you meet them.' Again, the wall of silence.

Nelly was half asleep, her chin on her knees. Maggie told Alex to push the car seats together for a bed. She spread a sleeping bag and quilt on the mattress for herself and Dayo and unbuttoned her shirt for the last feed of the evening. Alex looked away, made shy by Dayo's sucking, greedy pleasure. He remembered Ruth feeding Nelly at home while their father read to him. That had been long ago, when everything was normal.

Nelly and Dayo slept at once as though they hadn't a care in the world. Maggie glanced across at Alex. 'How old are you?' she asked.

'Sixteen.'

'Where are your parents?'

Alex told her, briefly.

'You don't say much, do you?' she asked.

That's funny, Alex thought. *I used to.*

'It's OK,' she said. She blew out the candle and they lay in the dark.

When at last Alex slept, he had terrible dreams. People were dragging Nelly away down endless flights of smelly concrete stairs. He stood at the top, watching, too frightened to go after her. In the dream she was screaming, begging him to help her, but he couldn't make himself move. He woke in the night to the sound of real screaming coming from somewhere above his head.

Six

They were late up next morning. Maggie warmed water on the stove – only a drop because she had to carry it up nine flights of stairs from a standpipe below. She let Nelly help her wash Dayo in a big basin. Dayo kicked her little fat legs and smiled her gummy smile and soaked both of them.

'Shall I get her clothes?' Nell asked when Dayo was dry.

Maggie nodded. 'Nappies are in the bag by the door.'

Nelly went and looked inside. 'There's only rags in there.'

'That's right. Disposables. Use 'em and chuck 'em. Clever, eh?'

Nelly nodded. Alex could see she was impressed.

'Breakfast now.' Alex had thought Maggie would never offer. 'Find it, I mean,' she said, and his heart sank.

There was a market down at the back of the flats where they picked up plums and an apple, three spuds and some wrinkly brown greens from underneath the back of the stalls. Alex had often seen beggars, doing just this. His face was red with shame, Nelly was horrified. An old man gave Maggie a bag of bread, stale but not mouldy. 'For the wee lassie,' he said. Somebody else was selling powdered milk.

'It's an awful price,' Maggie said, 'but I'll get some.'

They called at the rag stall and Maggie swapped the plums for a bag of rags. 'Pallets now, for the fire,' she said. Alex managed to find four and lugged them up the nine flights to the flat. When they got there, they found the door to Maggie's flat looked different. One hinge was broken and there were new marks on the battered paintwork.

Maggie handed Dayo to Alex. She took a knife from inside her coat and kicked the door open. Nothing happened. She leaned in a little way, still tensed to run if need be. Inside, the stove was gone, the chimney pipe, the sheets of tin. Everything else was smashed and dirtied. Whoever had done it had left.

Maggie sat down on the floor and cried, with her shoulders shaking, and tears and snot running down her face. Alex would have liked to make her a cup of tea, just for something to do, but there was no tea, no stove, and no cup.

Maggie stopped sobbing after a while, blew her nose on a rag and wiped her eyes.

'I'll go from here now,' she said. 'I should have gone before.'

'Where will you go?'

'I know a place outside the town. It's empty, but it's in good nick. It's over towards Gartbeg, but not so far. It'll do for a start.'

'Will you manage, on your own?'

'There's folk will help me. I knew something like this would happen some time, so I hid a few bits. Best pack up and go. You'd better come with me. No sense in being here when they come back.'

She went through to the smelly bathroom and wrenched the hardboard panel away from the side of the bath. She fished out a tin of baby milk, four tins of beans, a bag of oats, a pair of leather boots, a knife, a back pack and a roll of polythene.

Alex was starving and Nelly felt the same but she didn't even whimper about breakfast. Maggie changed Dayo's nappy. Nelly wouldn't use the loo, she said she'd rather go behind a bush later. Alex went, then wished he hadn't. When he tried to flush it, water gushed back up the pipe, overflowing the pan and running in a smelly stream across the bathroom floor.

Back in the other room, Maggie patted and petted Dayo back into her coat and slid her into her sling. She buckled her on in front and turned her back for Alex to heave the backpack up onto her shoulders. Then she pulled her hat well down, took Nelly by the hand, and looked for the last time round the flat. Alex saw tears in her eyes.

At the bottom of the cracked and stinking stairs there was a dog lying dead on its back with the bolt of a crossbow sticking out of its neck. Two lads squatted beside it. Alex recognised them from the group who'd chased him yesterday.

'Morning, Miss,' one said to Maggie, all good manners this time. 'What'll you give us for a piece o' meat?'

'It ain't yours to sell,' the other snapped. 'Your dad killed it. He'll kill you too if you sell it all!'

'It is mine too. It was my dog.'

'What's up wi' you?' the first one asked, looking at Maggie's face. 'Too good to eat dog meat? What do you live here for then?'

'I don't live here,' Maggie said. 'Not any more.'

'You do! You're the one wi' the stove.'

'What do you know about my stove you thieving little bastard?'

'Nothing. Keep your knickers on.'

'She don't wear knickers.'

'Ignorant wee turds,' Maggie snapped.

Both lads spat gobs of phlegm on the floor by Maggie's feet. Alex felt a spatter of stones on his back as they left the block.

'You shouldn't have said turds,' Nelly said primly.

'You're right,' Maggie replied. 'They probably still have the crossbow.'

They did about five miles without a rest, then sat down in a field with the hedge between them and the road and shared a can of beans from the tin.

'What's it like, where we're going?' Nelly asked.

'It's just an empty croft with heather all round it. I saw it once when I was out walking with Moyo. We used to say we'd go and live there, once his studying was over. And now I am. But not with him.'

'Is it far?'

'Yes. But you're doing fine.'

It was evening when they turned off the small back road onto an even smaller track. Maggie carried the backpack as well as Dayo and Nelly clung to Alex's back with her hands under his chin, half strangling him. As far as Alex could tell, they were still heading for Gartbeg. He and Nelly could stay with Maggie for one night and go on in the morning. He wasn't too sure of the route any more, but west would take him to the coast, he knew that much.

The sun was going down red and the air was damp and cool. The track led downhill, and a burn ran beside it with a little mist rising along its course. The house was tiny, with a straggling bit of garden behind a low stone wall. The burn ran right by the back door. In front there were two stunted fruit trees. The windows were small, with rags of curtains hanging in them, but none of the glass was broken. The roof was made of slates and one or two had blown off, but it didn't look too bad.

Maggie strode down the slope in her thick boots as though she owned the place and rattled the door – which was locked, of course. Down on the doorstep stood a pot of dead ferns. Maggie tilted it to one side: underneath were about five hundred woodlice and a key. Scratched in charcoal on the bottom of the flowerpot a tiny pin man danced.

'Why do folks bother with locking doors,' she asked,

'when they hide the key where any fool can find it?'

'Who drew that picture?' Nelly asked. 'That little dancing man?'

'I don't know who drew it. But I know what it means. It means we should be safe here,' Maggie answered.

She unlocked the door and they stood still, Maggie with Dayo on her back, Alex holding Nelly by the hand, and listened. Nothing. The house breathed out a damp and musty smell. The quiet was profound. The burn sang behind the house and the wind combed the heather on the hill with a gentle hush hush sough.

A little whirl of dust flew up off the step. Inside they could see a bare room, a scrubbed table, no sign of habitation. And yet. They stood together looking in uncertainly, waiting. Sure enough, after a few moments the occupants of the house stepped out through the front door, stopped still on the doorstep, cocked their heads on one side and looked up from out of cold, round eyes.

'*Twa Corbies*,' Maggie whispered. '*Where shall we gang and dine the day?*' She shook her head and laughed quietly with relief. 'You two stay outside. Here, Alex. Take Dayo for me. I'll go in on my own and see what they've been dining on.'

'What do you mean, *twa corbies*?' Alex asked. 'What are you talking about, Maggie?'

'It's an old song, about the two crows – they're going to have their supper off a new-killed knight lying beside the road. *Ye'll sit on his white hause-bane, And I'll pike out his bonny blue e'en.* It used to make me shiver, when I was a wee lass.'

Alex held Dayo and Maggie stepped over the sill. The crows took off in a clatter, their black feathers glinting like oil in the evening sun. As they flew over the apple tree, Alex looked up and saw them turn their heads in slow unison to look down at him. One croaked to the other. Then they flew over the hill and were gone.

Maggie's boots clumped noisily across the stone floors of the two rooms downstairs, thumped up the stairs, entered each of the two bedrooms and clumped back down.

'It's OK,' she called. 'They were just feedin' on an old dead rabbit. I was afraid it might be something more.'

The remains of the rabbit – white bones and a few balls of grey fur – were scattered on the floor. A broken window showed where the crows had got in to feed on it.

'Did they bring the rabbit in here?' Nelly asked.

'Aye. Maybe. Or maybe someone else did, and left a bit behind. Corbies can smell a dead thing. We'll clear away what's left of the creature. You find firewood, Alex. Then get some apples from out the front if you can find any. Nelly, you can help me look for tatties in the garden at the back.'

They had potatoes baked in the grate for supper, eaten by firelight, with shrivelled little apples for pudding. When the food was gone, and Dayo had been fed and changed, Maggie asked Alex which bedroom he and Nelly wanted.

'I don't want a bedroom,' Nelly said quickly, before Alex could answer. 'I want us to stay together. Down here. By the fire.'

'I'd like that fine myself,' Maggie replied. 'Alex? Is that all right with you?'

Alex nodded. He had come to dread sleeping; the fears he managed to control by day rose up by night and filled his dreams with horror. So they lay down to sleep in a row on the tattered rug in front of the fire, with Maggie at one end and Alex at the other. They'd taken blankets off the beds upstairs and rolled themselves in these.

Alex woke in the night, because an owl was hunting close by. He put a bit more wood on the fire and lay awake thinking about his parents. Then the face of the dying prisoner came into his mind and stayed there, looking at him.

Next morning, Maggie gave Alex what food she could spare. 'Head for where the sun goes down,' she said. 'I think you've to cross the hills before you come to Gartbeg. There's a lot of woods, pine trees an' that. When you come out the other side you'll see the sea. I think your Gran's house will be quite close by then.'

'Will we be there tomorrow night?' Nelly asked.

'No, pet. I doubt it. It's not so far, but it's rough going. You'll have to find somewhere to sleep tonight. Get inside a sheep pen or a barn or something. Make sure it's got a door you can shut. Don't try a house on your own, not even if you think it's empty. Not unless someone's drawn a wee pin man on the door.'

'What does that pin man mean?' Alex asked again.

'*Good folk* is all it means. Don't fret. You'll reach your granny's house. You'll find your parents, or else they'll find you.'

'What about you?' Nelly asked. 'Will you find Dayo's dad?'

'I don't think so. But I'll keep his wee girl safe and well.'

Alex found it hard to part from Maggie. Her pride in coping and her belief that somehow she and Dayo would survive, made him feel braver too.

Seven

Ruth and Rob lay in the dark, touching but not able to hold hands because they were still handcuffed. The floor they lay on was cold and it smelled bad. There were no sounds of breathing or of groaning any more. Whoever else had been in the cell with them must have been taken away while they slept.

Ruth moved her head slightly to whisper in Rob's ear. 'D'you think Alex and Nell are safe? D'you think they've got there yet?'

'I'm sure they haven't caught them, love,' Rob whispered back. 'If they had, they'd have let us know. If they tell us they have, we mustn't believe them. Not unless they can prove it. OK, Ruth?'

'OK.'

'Alex'll make it. He'll look after Nelly.'

They lay still for a while, they eyes getting used to

the dark. There was a grating up above them, and a little dirty light came through. Street light, not sunlight. So it must be night time. Somebody yelled, a sound of anger, somewhere close at hand. Somebody laughed. Ruth rolled slightly over so that she could feel Rob's warmth the length of her body.

'They won't leave us together,' Rob said. 'Not for long. If they question you first, make them contact Dandy. I'll do the same if they start with me. That way he'll know that we need help. Meanwhile we can tell them whatever they want to know about Road Sickness, if they ask us. They'll probably ask you. They must know you're a doctor. I'll talk about the road, the contaminated materials, but I'll tell them the foreman didn't know we were taking samples. We can say that Dandy gave us petrol because he thought we had permits to visit Mum – we can say we lied about it. Tell them to get in touch with him and ask. I'll do the same. OK?'

'OK.'

'We won't be in here long. Dandy will get us out.'

'I know. I'm not scared about us. I'm scared about Alex and Nelly.'

'They're safe. I'm sure of it. Alex will get them both to Gartbeg. Dandy will take over once they get there.

They're safe. I know they are. Don't cry, Ruth. Don't cry.'

A voice, frightened this time, not angry, echoed down from above. Ruth pressed her face against Rob's neck. The two of them lay still and quiet on the wet floor, pale light from the grating overhead outlining their dark shapes. Footsteps approached, clattering down a flight of steps. They stopped outside the cell door and the bolt slid back.

★ ★ ★

Alex and Nelly walked west all day, as far as Alex could judge. Nelly plodded beside him with her head down and her hand in his and when they talked, they talked about how things used to be – times they'd enjoyed, like birthdays. Christmases. Good times with their uncle Dandy. Every now and then Alex would haul his sister up on to his back and carry her. Each time he did, she slept. When he felt he must rest, he'd lower her gently back down and she would wake, and walk on, uncomplaining. Now and then she cried, but silently. Alex could only tell when he saw tears dripping off her chin.

Gradually, as the evening closed in, both of them grew afraid. They were high up now, on top of the hills that Alex had been heading for. They couldn't see the house by the burn when they looked back; it was folded away between blue ridges they had trudged over. They couldn't see the sea in front either, because of mist and storm blowing in from the west. Alex knew that there would be no barn or farm building so high up. Only, perhaps, a walkers' hut.

Now and then the wind rattled the gorse that grew beside their path. Once a black grouse got up almost from under their feet, making them jump out of their skins. They saw no people. Alex expected to see deer, and told Nelly to look out for them, hoping to cheer her up. But something must have scared them off because they saw none, though it was good deer country. They found themselves stopping as they climbed, to look behind them and to search the countryside all round. They saw nothing but heather, with occasional shoulders of lichened rock pushing up through the peat coat of the land. Alex glanced back over his shoulder often. Presently Nelly tugged his hand and stood still, frowning.

'Something's behind us, Alex. I can feel it.'

'There's nobody out here, Nelly. Only us.'

'I don't mean people.'

They stood still, listening, afraid of what they'd hear. Faint behind, rising from the valley they had left they heard the first deep call. Nelly tightened her grip on

Alex's hand and they stared back down the hillside where the path wound down, empty, a trail worn white in the sandy soil between the heather and the gorse. The deep, baying call came again. Then silence. Long, wind-blown, out-under-the-sky silence. Suddenly, a dreadful choir called back, hunting voices tearing up the silence, answering that one, deep voice. Alex felt the hair on his scalp rise.

'It's wolves, Alex.'

Howling arose close by, near and getting nearer. 'It's dogs, Nelly. Coming this way.'

'They're coming after us, Alex!'

There was no tree to scramble into, no door to bolt, no stair to climb. Nothing to do but run. They threw themselves up the hillside, running without knowing where they were running to, just running, anywhere, so long as it would save them from the sound that swelled behind them, the hungry, hunting sound.

At first fear gave Nelly speed. Her small feet hardly seemed to touch the heather, but the yip and holler of the hunting dogs grew closer. They were gaining. Nelly began to trip and stumble, slowing Alex until it took all his strength and courage not to run ahead and leave her. He swung her up onto his back without pausing and ran on, faster now. It was Nelly who saw the shelter

71

first and pointed, shouting in his ear. The rock pile looked like part of the hillside from a distance. Close to, they saw great slabs of granite piled on one another like plates and bowls. Behind, but closing fast, the leader of the pack broke cover and hurled himself at Alex, big-footed, heavy-jawed, nose down and red tongue lolling, so close Alex could smell his breath. Shoving Nelly ahead of him, blind with panic, Alex found a narrow gap between two massive rocks. He pushed Nelly ahead and jammed in after her, then turned to hammer with his boots at two blades of rock that leaned inwards precariously on either side of the gap.

He kicked furiously at the bottom of one and felt it shift. He kicked again, harder, and the rocks fell in, one across the other, blocking the entrance to the crack just as the lead dog's head pushed in. The dog struggled free, bringing a fall of rocks and pebbles crashing down behind it. Then it began to scrabble, worrying at the rock. The pack would have trouble digging in – but Alex could see that he and Nelly would never dig out. He squeezed past Nelly and began to wriggle backwards, pulling her behind him. He could feel the rock opening up on each side of him. He struggled to turn round, scraping knees and elbows, and pushed through into the bottom of a tall chimney of rock. Nelly followed. A peal of thunder ripped down from the sky. Nelly crouched low, eyes shut, ears blocked. Alex put his arms round her and squeezed.

'Nelly,' he said. 'We've got to climb up high where they can't get us. Just in case they manage to break through.' They could hear the odd rumble of thunder, and in between, snarling and panting and the sound of digging paws. They smelled the heavy stink of wet dog. Wild dogs. The kind Donald had warned them of. A little light came filtering down from above. Alex could see climbing places. There was a sort of shelf, halfway up the chimney. He tugged at Nelly, pointed, finger on lips, pushed her up ahead of him, making her stand on his shoulders, then climbed up behind her, waiting, muscles shaking, while she inched the next way up. Finally they were both sitting on the ledge, with their backs to the rock and their feet drawn up. Alex did not think the dogs could climb so high. He slumped, one arm round Nelly, and they clung together silently. At last, after what felt like hours, they heard the dogs move off, their disappointment loud in the quiet of the evening.

The panting woke him. The cave was lit softly with dawn sunlight filtered through cloud. Alex felt Nelly stiffen as she woke and a warm trickle reached his leg.

'Alex. I've wet myself.'

'Never mind. It doesn't matter.'

'What is it, Alex?'

'Dog. Outside. Don't worry. It can't get us up here.'

The panting stopped, then started, loud and gusty.

'Let's wait until it's gone, Alex.'

'You wait. You're safe here, Nell. I'll try to get out at the top and look down.'

Alex jammed toes and elbows into chinks and cracks, hauling himself slowly up the chimney of rock, an inch at a time. Below on the shelf Nelly waited, cold and clammy.

'What is it, Alex?' she called softly, when he'd disappeared. 'What can you see?'

Alex could see a dog, big, dirty and thin, with a rough coat. He wore a heavy leather collar, the kind with studs on. There was a ring in his collar from which a chain dangled. The rest of the chain trailed on the ground in a tangle of sticks and broken branches; the end was snagged round a tooth of rock. The dog shifted his head and the chain jerked taut. He grunted and dropped his head. Alex could see the rusty stain of old blood round his neck. A little trickle of fresh red seeped out from underneath his collar.

A tiny sound behind him made Alex jump and swivel. It was Nelly, emerging like a chimney sweep at his back. The dog rumbled deep in his chest: *keep away*! and put his front paws on the base of the rock tower. The chain snagged again, the dog yelped and twisted his head. He put one paw up to scratch at his collar, whining. A raw patch showed under the heavy leather.

'He's hurting,' Nelly whispered.

'I know.'

'You'll have to get his collar off.'

'I can't.'

'I've got some of Ludo's chews in my pocket. You could give him those.'

Reluctantly, Alex clambered a few feet down towards the dog. Alone, without the pack, his growl was only bluster.

'Good dog,' Alex said softly. 'Good old boy.'

He dropped a chew down and the old dog nosed it, flicked it into his mouth with a long tongue, swallowed, and looked up expectantly.

'You're supposed to chew them,' Nelly said. 'That's why they're called chews.'

'He's starving, Nell. I bet he can't hunt with that chain on.'

Alex fixed the dog with a severe look and said 'Sit!' Nothing happened.

'Try *drop* instead of *sit*. Some people teach their dogs that, Alex.'

Alex fixed him with another severe look. '*Drop!*' he ordered. The old dog sat back on his haunches and smiled. Alex threw him a chew. 'Good dog. Good old boy.'

He climbed down the last few feet, talking gently to the old dog all the while. The dog was frightened now, but Alex had told him to drop, so he stayed put. Alex jumped softly onto the heather beside him, bent down and undid his collar. It was disgusting: crusted with dried blood, stinking of pain and infection. It fell on the ground and Alex kicked it away. The dog's plumed tail flicked slowly, experimentally, from side to side.

'Good old boy,' Nelly said, only now leaving the safety of the rock tower. 'That's better, isn't it?' She held out the last chew and the dog swallowed it whole. Then he sat back on his haunches so that his face was on a level with Nelly's and looked at her expectantly.

'No more,' Nelly told him. 'Sorry.'

The dog got up, shook himself slowly, testing to see if the pain was going to return. When it didn't, he shook himself more vigorously. Then he trotted away down to a puddle of rain water, drank, looked back once over his shoulder, and headed off the way the pack had left.

The storm was over and the sky was light behind Alex and Nelly. Ahead in the west the land was still black. Alex thought of the hidden sea beyond the land. It lay, rough, cold and deep, with nothing but a few islands between this coast and Newfoundland. He thought of his mum and dad, somewhere behind him now. *We're surviving*, he told them. *You survive too*.

'What d'you think Ludo would have done if he'd come face to face with that dog, Nelly?' he asked.

'Same as I did when we heard it panting, probably,' she said.

'Are you drying out?'

She nodded.

'We'd better go on.'

Eight

Alex and Nelly scrambled down the hill into the valley beyond. Tall tufts of rushes and vivid green hillocks of moss showed where the ground was wettest. An old path wound round, finding out the drier patches. They walked in all the boggy places, hoping the water would cover their scent. They stopped and listened often, dreading the sound of hunting dogs behind them, but heard only the cry of a curlew, and now and then the whirr of grouse. They walked all morning, following the valley west. In the afternoon they climbed out, crossed a low ridge with straggling, wind-bent pine trees, and found themselves above a wide belt of forest, black under the red of sunset. It lay blocking their path west. They would have to go through it to get to the coast.

'What horrible trees,' Nelly said. 'It looks haunted. Like the kind of forest where you get wolves and vampires.'

'It's just a forest,' Alex snapped. 'Pine trees, planted in rows. There are no wolves and vampires. You're in Scotland, stupid. Not Transylvania.'

The look of the trees scared him as well. They looked unfriendly. Regimented. Dark. Gravel paths ran in unnaturally straight lines through them. Black dark shadow lapped each path like inky water.

'There are wild dogs,' Nelly persisted. 'There could be wolves. And witches. There could be anything. You don't know.'

'We've got to go through it anyway, to get to Gran's. So shut up.'

'What if we're not out the other side by the time it gets dark?'

'We'll sleep in there and go on in the morning.'

'If we do,' Nelly said, 'I'm sleeping up a tree.'

Once they got in under the trees the light faded and everything grew silent. Their feet on the path made too loud a sound; they crept onto the edge where grass straggled and walked carefully. All they could hear were their own footfalls, soft on the fallen pine needles, and sometimes a crack when one of them stepped on a stick. Alex felt watched, though he couldn't say who – or what – was watching him.

He found himself thinking of a story that had been

going round school before he left – one of those stupid stories people tell each other, not believing them. He wished now that he hadn't listened. Some kid had found his dog gnawing strange bones, apparently. Long bones. He couldn't think of anything with bones like that. He showed them to his dad and his dad said they looked human. This boy and his dad thought maybe his dog had been digging in the cemetery nearby so they went to take a look. None of the graves had been disturbed. But they found a place where there had been a fire, and people camping out.

That was common enough. People fell out of the bottom of Beta Sector all the time. You only had to lose your job, or fail to pay your rent. Most of them went on the road, camping out where ever they found open ground. If you fell far enough, you turned into a runner. Otherwise you put up a shack and stayed until police or the army moved you on. With so many people homeless, every city had its shanty towns and every shanty town its outer ring of dugouts and tarpaulins, fires of rubbish and old car tyres, markets where shanty folk bartered for things that others threw away. Everyone told stories of the shanty folk and the runners. They lived on dope, killed anyone who strayed onto their manor.

Anyway, this boy's dog went running over to the ashes of the camp fire, down between the grave stones, tail wagging, and came back with more bones. Long bones. There was a pile of clothes beside the fire, the boy said. Shoes. Odds and ends. And two round skulls. The point of the story was that shanty folk – beggars and vagrants and so on – had put themselves outside human society. They had begun to eat each other.

A story, Alex told himself. A stupid story. Round him, the forest was filling up with evening noises; little stops and starts of sound that could not be explained. A forest is like an old house on a quiet evening. You hear footsteps where nobody is walking. Coming out of silence, each noise seems significant. Just one dead twig, falling from where it has been caught between two living ones, will make you jump when it hits the ground. Alex had been hearing padding, the odd breath, a crack now and then, for some time – hearing it and not hearing it, because he didn't want to. Nelly reached up and took his hand. Maybe she'd heard it too. When the shot rang out, both of them froze.

Two snappy little terriers came bouncing through the wood, one with a wood pigeon still flapping in its mouth. One stepped out into the path in front of them, the other slipped round behind and dropped onto its stumpy tail. There was a metallic click and Alex realised that someone had stepped onto the path behind him. He wondered if the click meant there was a gun pointed at his back. He turned his head, slowly, to see.

The girl on the path wore a man's heavy jacket with a belt round the middle. Two rabbits and a pigeon dangled from the belt. Her face was very brown, as though she lived outside, and her tufty hair looked as though she'd cut it herself. She had dark, feathery eyebrows and blue eyes. She was beautiful. That was the first thing Alex noticed. The second was that her gun was only a shotgun, but it was pointed at his chest.

'Where are you off to, through the wood?' she asked.

Nelly pressed tight against Alex, her finger nails digging into his hand. Alex found he couldn't answer, because of the gun pointing at his chest.

'What are you doing here?' the girl asked.

'Put the gun down,' Alex said, and to his surprise, she did. 'We're on our way to Gartbeg. On the coast.'

'What's at Gartbeg?'

'Our granny is. We're going to visit her. Because she's hurt her back,' Nell added.

'Off to see your granny? Just like little red riding hood. And you met my wolf,' the girl said, smiling.

'That's not a wolf,' Nell said. 'It's a dog. Make it get off the path.'

The girl whistled and both dogs trotted over to sit behind her. She took the pigeon, wrung its neck quickly, and hung it from her belt.

'That better?' she asked. Nell nodded. 'My name's Anna. What's yours?'

'Nelly.'

'I'm Alex.'

'Are you on your own?' Anna asked. 'Just the two of you?' Alex nodded.

'Well you'd better come with me now you've seen me,' she said. 'My mum'll feed you. You look hungry.'

'We are,' Nelly agreed. 'Very.'

'We can't. We have to get on,' Alex said.

Anna shook her head. 'Sorry,' she said. 'I can't let you go.'

'Why not?'

'There are soldiers coming. They're on the far side of the forest now. But you're practically on top of our camp. You could lead them onto us without even knowing it.'

'Who's at your camp?'

'You'll see.'

Alex and Nelly walked ahead of her. She followed

with her gun. Both dogs stayed close until, just as it was getting too dark to see where they were putting their feet, a light twinkled ahead and the terriers ran on, barking as dogs do among friends.

Alex saw that they had reached a clearing in the trees. A small fire burned and about a dozen people, men and women, black and white, sat round it, eating from a big open pot that stood in the raked-out embers. A plump and dirt-smudged baby snored softly on a young man's lap. A toddler cuddled into the crook of someone's arm, waiting for the spoon to find his mouth. *Runners*, Alex thought. *These are the runners.*

Everyone looked up as Anna, Alex and Nelly stepped into the clearing. One of the women jumped up and hurried over. She kissed Anna, glanced at Alex and smiled down at Nelly. 'Who's this you've brought back, Anna?' she enquired.

'There's soldiers on the far side of the forest, Mum. I thought I'd better bring them in.'

'Quite right.'

Alex introduced himself and Nelly. The woman's name was Brigid. She was Anna's mother, and also, it seemed to Alex, something of a leader among the people gathered round the fire. 'Come over by the fire you two,' she said, 'where we can see you. Don't be frightened. If you're not enemies to us, we're none to you.'

Alex held Nelly's hand and together they joined the people in the firelight. Beyond, a couple of ponies, tethered in the shadows, stamped and snorted. Dogs snouted for fleas. A rich, sweet smell drifted from pot and fire towards Alex, making his mouth water.

'Sit down,' Brigid said. 'Food first. Questions after.'

Alex and Nelly sat, staring at the pot. Nelly was white and quiet, leaning close to Alex. Brigid ladled food from the pot into a plastic bowl, stuck two spoons in and handed it to Alex. Someone passed round hot tin mugs of tea with no milk. Anna sat between her mother, Brigid, and Madoc, her father. Madoc was big and old and weather-beaten. He smoothed Anna's short hair and her brown forehead, then shook her gently.

'We were worried, pet,' he said. 'Will brought news of the soldiers. We didn't know if you'd have seen them before they saw you.'

'I was OK, Dad. They're noisy. I saw them, and went the other way.'

Nelly finished eating and put her head down on Alex's legs. Her thumb crept up to her mouth and her eyes rolled shut.

'Time to answer a few questions, son,' Madoc told Alex, when he too had finished. 'Once we know a bit about you, we'll maybe find you somewhere safe to stay. If you need a place, that is.'

'You're runners, aren't you?' Alex asked. Madoc nodded. Suddenly, Alex was too tired to lie. Something told him to trust Anna. And if he trusted Anna, he must trust the runners. He shifted Nelly gently, stretched his hands to the warmth, and told his story to the dirty, weathered faces round the fire. He began with the dying prisoner on the high white bed in his mother's clean hospital, and ended with his grandmother's house at Gartbeg by the sea, where his parents might now be waiting, worried sick.

'We know about the sickness on the road,' Madoc said, when Alex had finished. 'Foreman's a friend of ours. But you can't go to Gartbeg now.'

'Why not?'

'Because the police may be there. Waiting for you.'

'I don't think so. I think my uncle Dandy will have sorted it all out by now.'

Madoc shrugged. 'He may have. And he may not. They wanted you back at Stepgavie, where the old man let the sheep out and you ran.'

'We have to go there. It's the only way Mum and

Dad will find us. Dandy can fix anything. He'll tell the police to let them go and they will. They'll go to gran's house to look for us. We have to be there.'

Madoc shook his head. 'Go if you must, but stay with us a night or two. Rest up and find your feet. Runners will help you, if you meet them. But be careful, son.'

Alex was silent. He didn't want to think about anything any more. He wanted to sleep.

Talk shifted to the police and the soldiers and this or that person who had been taken, or escaped. Alex slept, while voices came and went around him. He woke to a new face, bending low over him. Long hair tied back. A bushy beard. A gentle face, lined, tired, weathered down like leather.

'Wake up, Alex. I want to talk to you. I was there when your mum and dad were taken. They're all right. I was watching and I know what happened to them after.'

Alex sat up. He found that he could hardly breathe. Fear must have shown on his face because the man put a hand on his shoulder.

'Don't worry son. They're prisoners. But they're alive.'

'Have you spoken to them?' Alex asked.

The man shook his head. 'Not yet. But we can get a message to them, more than likely. Brigid told me to wake you, just to let you know they're OK. Go back to sleep now. We'll be moving on tomorrow.'

Just before dawn Anna shook Alex awake. 'Get up!' she hissed. 'Soldiers are coming. Wake Nelly up. Grab anything you brought here. Quick!'

Within minutes the clearing was empty. Turf covered the fire and a little line of people, dogs and horses stood in the fuzzy dawn light with Madoc at the front and Brigid at the back. Brigid pushed the rope leads of two dogs into Nelly's hand, heaved a sack of supplies over her shoulder, and lifted a toddler onto Alex's back.

The light grew brighter. They moved off fast, pushing between trees, over and round fallen timber, deeper and deeper into the wood. The baby they'd seen asleep on his father's lap the night before gave in to the joggle of hurrying feet and dozed again, his round head bouncing on his mother's back. Alex's toddler clung tight round his neck and hummed into his ear. Anna walked next to Alex but they did not talk. Nell trotted in front, towed along by the dogs. Baggage was shifted from one of the ponies and a woman was heaved onto its back, all with hardly a break in the animal's stride.

After what felt like hours Will, the man who'd woken Alex in the night, ran up from behind. His brown face shone with sweat; it trickled down and disappeared into his bushy beard. He spoke urgently to Brigid who signalled a halt. Everybody stopped and sat, all in one movement. Up and down the path people eased packs off backs, adjusted boots, rubbed aching shoulders. Nelly pressed against Alex. The tired toddler slumped into his lap.

'What's happening?' he asked Anna. 'Why have we stopped?'

'It's Will,' she said. 'He's been watching the soldiers to see how close they are.'

'Are they chasing us?' Nelly asked.

Anna nodded.

'What will happen if they catch us?'

Will spoke briefly. 'They won't. Brigid and me are going back to see to 'em. The rest of you go on.'

There was no discussion. Alex felt a tug on his coat and looked down. The toddler was asking to be lifted back onto his shoulders. Alex lifted him.

'Alex,' Nelly whispered. 'Don't let me get left behind. I can't run much further.'

'You're doing great,' he said. 'You won't get left behind.'

'Wait for me Alex, if I do.'

'Of course I will, Nelly.'

'You can sit on my shoulders, Nelly, when you're tired,' Anna offered.

They started going uphill and soon slowed to a plod. The child on Alex's back clung doggedly. Nelly stumbled along, one hand on the lead Brigid had given her, the other hand in Alex's. Eventually they came to a place where patches of rock broke through the pine needles. There was short grass and a stream. Packs and bundles and sleepy kids were lowered to the ground.

'My feet hurt, Nelly.' Alex flopped onto the ground. 'See if you can get my boots off.' His socks were wet with blister burst and blood.

'I could get water in a mug,' Nell offered. Alex nodded. He sat with his eyes shut. Nelly fetched his water first, then some for the child in his lap, then some for herself. When she sat down she allowed Anna to soothe her battered feet with cold water.

Once darkness fell a fire was built and lit, food was produced. The tethered ponies moved in circles, grazing. Smoke drifted under the trees. Alex thought of Moyo. Was he perhaps safe, somewhere, sitting by a fire like this? If he was, would Maggie ever find him? There was no sign of Brigid or Will.

'They'll be back tomorrow,' Anna said. 'They'll wait to make sure they're not being followed.' She unrolled blankets for Nelly and they tucked her in with the toddler Alex had been carrying, whose name was The Minnow. The Minnow didn't seem to have an adult of his own.

'Don't go away while I'm asleep, Alex,' Nelly said.

'I'm not. I won't.'

She was asleep before he finished speaking.

Anna and Alex sat outside the ring of firelight, close enough to Nelly and The Minnow so that they could hear them if they woke and cried. It wasn't cold, but they could feel the autumn coming. The leaves overhead had a papery sound to their rustle though they were not yet yellow, and there was a pleasant leaf-mould smell behind the sting of wood smoke. A huge moon rose, pillowed in deep rich blue and with a border of sharp black leaves edging its russet face.

'Are you scared for your mother?' Alex asked. 'When she's away from you?'

'We're always scared about each other. All the time.'

'Me too. They pushed my mother over. She was crying. I can't stop thinking about her.'

'I had a friend who was caught. She was put on the roads this time last year.'

'A prisoner, you mean?'

Anna nodded.

'What had she done?'

'What planet did you live on, Alex? Before you fell off? You don't need to have *done* anything, to be put on the roads.'

Alex blushed. 'I thought it was a punishment. For breaking the law.'

'It is. But you can take your pick what you're being punished for. My friend was punished for being homeless. Or maybe for not working. Or else for being on the move without a permit. No job, no money. No money, no home. No home, no job. No job, move on. That's the way it goes. You don't know much about that, do you?' Alex shook his head.

'It's OK. I don't blame you. Most people don't. Until it happens to them. Or someone they know. *They* don't want you to know.'

'Is she still on the roads? Your friend?'

'No.'

'She got away?'

'Sort of. She's dead.'

'What's it like when somebody you know dies?' Alex asked.

'It's as if they're in another room. You can't get in and they can't get out. As you go on, there are more people in there. One day you'll be the only one left outside.'

They sat quietly for a while, close but not touching. Sometimes you know, when you meet someone, that all things might be possible between you, if life will let you stay together. Passion. Or love. Between you stands the empty house of the future. Perhaps you'll enter it together. Perhaps not.

Presently they spread their sleeping bags beside Nelly and The Minnow and lay down back to back. Alex would have liked to put his arms round Anna and hold her all night. But he didn't, and they both dropped into sleep.

When they woke in the morning, Brigid and Will were there. Will's right arm stuck out of his bloody sleeve and he was hardly conscious. Anna was up and beginning to cut his coat away ready to wash his wound. The thought of what might be happening to his parents flooded Alex's mind like cold, dirty water and he rolled over in his blanket, crying.

'Why are you crying, Alex?' Nelly asked.

'I'm not.'

'You are.'

'I'm worried. About Mum and Dad.'

'Why are they prisoners, Alex?' Nell asked.

'I thought you were asleep when Will told me.'

'Why, Alex?'

'I don't know. Maybe for taking samples of the gravel.'

'What are we going to do?'

'Go to Gartbeg. To Granny.'

'What if the police are there? Like Madoc said.'

'We'll be careful. Maybe they won't be. Maybe Dandy will have sorted them out.'

'I want to stay here. With Anna and the others. I don't want to go on with just you, Alex. I don't like it, when it's just us.'

'I know. But we have to go. When Mum and Dad come looking for us, we have to be there.'

'I'll walk a mile or two with you,' Anna offered, when she'd dressed Will's arm. 'I'll see you onto the right track.'

★ ★ ★

94

When it was time for Anna to turn back, and Alex and Nelly to go on alone, they stopped on the grassy path and Nelly took Alex's hand. She held it tightly, looking from her brother's face to Anna's without speaking. Neither Alex nor Anna wanted to be the first to say goodbye and turn away. In the end, Alex found the courage to lean forward and kiss Anna. Anna put her hands to his face, smiling but sad. She bent and kissed Nelly's grubby cheek.

'Goodbye,' she said. 'Keep out of that other room.'

★ ★ ★

The road surface was greasy with mud and it was hard to keep upright. Ruth got to her knees. Sweat ran into her eyes making them sting. Her back was on fire.

'Keep it steady,' the woman behind her muttered. 'Slow and steady. That way you won't fall so often.'

Cars flicked by just feet away from where the prisoners worked, drenching them over and over with muddy water. Lorries roared by so close they shook the ground. The mountain of sub-base Ruth was shovelling seemed to grow, not shrink. Red dust splashed up over her hands, her feet, her face. She glanced across to where Rob worked, bent double, prying up loose tarmac with a swinging pick. New bruising on his face looked dark in the shadows cast by the tower lights. He glanced over, caught her eye and smiled.

If we knew Alex and Nelly were safe, Ruth thought, *if we knew they were safe, we could bear this.*

Nine

Kate Kentigern was an unusual grandmother. Tall and commanding, her white hair sleek in tied-back plaits, she smelled of turpentine and pipe tobacco. She painted every day, wearing an overall smeared with oil paint and other unidentifiable substances. Each time she stood back from her easel to consider her work she would light her pipe and send a shower of ash and matches down onto the floor. Watching her as a little boy, Alex had feared she might catch fire.

Kate Kentigern could cook, although she didn't like to. Staying with her made mealtimes a constant surprise. But she made good bread, and kept a goat for milk and cheese. She grew what vegetables she could. Beyond that, food was a mystery to her. 'Why cook it when it's better raw?' she'd say, slapping down bread, cheese and salad. The only things Kate couldn't do without were whisky in the evening, and tobacco all day.

She liked to look at things. She kept a magnifying glass on the kitchen windowsill beside a pair of binoculars. With the binoculars she watched birds fly, clouds come and go, weather off the sea, the rise and fall of tides. When Nelly was new-born, paying her first visit to her grandmother, Kate had fetched the magnifying glass and pored over her, examining minutely her silk-soft skin, her fine eyebrows, her milky, all-seeing eyes.

With Alex, her first grandchild, she felt more at ease than she had ever felt with her own warring, jealous boys, Dandy and Rob. With Alex, Kate Kentigern felt, from the beginning, at home, companionable. She loved and admired him without feeling that she had to teach him anything. And he loved her, wholeheartedly.

Thinking about his grandmother, Alex let himself relax. He let his mind float free. It floated mostly towards Anna. She knew about things he'd never even thought about. Soldiers. Wringing pigeons' necks. Dressing wounds. But she hadn't minded when he kissed her. She could have pulled back, but she didn't. He would see her again. Somehow, he'd find her. And then . . . and then Nelly broke into his little dream castle and sent it crashing with a load of questions.

'Alex, does Granny Kate know we're coming?'

'No.'

'Will she be pleased to see us?'

'Yes. Of course she will. She always is, Nelly.'

'What if the police are there. Like Brigid said, Alex.'

'Then I don't know. Gran will know what to do. Or Dandy will.'

'Alex, do you think Ludo's OK?'

'I've got no idea. I expect so.'

'I bet he's missing me.'

'I bet he's not missing your hat.'

'He likes my hat.'

'Does not.'

'Does.'

'Shush, Nelly.'

'Why?'

'Shut up. I heard something.'

'Alex . . .' Nelly whispered. 'I can *smell* something.'

Alex pulled Nelly off the path and back under some overhanging bushes. They crouched together, listening. Both of them could smell old dirt and tobacco. Neither of them spoke or moved. A ragged figure stepped out from behind a stone wall and stood in the middle of the path. Alex could tell by the way he stood blocking the path that he knew they were there. Keeping his eye on the ragged man, Alex drew Nelly gently backwards, away from the path. He longed to turn and bolt, but he dared not take his eyes off that dark figure. So he did not see the man and woman waiting quietly behind him and Nelly, tucked in under a clump of holly bushes. The first he knew of them was when the man stepped out and grabbed him, twisting his arms up behind his back. The woman grabbed Nelly and hauled her out onto the path, one hand across her mouth to stifle her scream. Alex followed, arms twisted tight and painful.

All three of their captors were creased, grimed, wrinkled and layered with dirt. Even their faces were the colour of mud. Their hair was like matted felt, hanging down in greasy hanks. They didn't speak, not even to each other. They marched off, the woman lifting Nell half off her feet, away from the path, up past the hollies and through a prickly thicket that formed a kind of barricade. Behind it leaned a shack made of stones and turf with a flapping piece of canvas for a door.

There was a fire in front of the shack, and a black pot balanced on two stones. One of the men pulled some lengths of stinking bandage from his pocket and tied one tightly round Nell's mouth. Her eyes looked out above it, terrified. He tied her wrists behind her back, and her ankles together. Then he did the same to Alex.

The woman pulled a dead rabbit out of her deep coat pocket. She took a knife from her belt and began to paunch and skin it. She jointed the body and tossed the bits into the pot. She threw the intestines and skin on the fire.

'Coney for starters. What for afters?' she remarked to the men, who laughed. 'Can't see anybody giving much for them two. May as well go in the pot.'

'Depends who wants 'em,' the man replied. 'Could be good money there.'

'Two little Alpha Sector chickens. Not quite so pretty as they once was, but you can tell. Couldn't do a day's work if you beat 'em black and blue. Who's goin' to pay good money for that?'

'Use yer loaf,' the second man grunted. 'Wasn't we told to keep an eye out for two Alpha kids?'

The first man smiled and nodded. 'Hand 'em over to the boys in blue and pick up what they give us.'

Everyone fell silent again.

After a while they pulled the pot off the fire and ate from it, dipping spoons in. They gave Alex and Nell nothing. They passed a bottle round and round till it was empty and then they bundled into the shack and began to snore.

Nell was crying silently. Alex wriggled over to her

101

like a caterpillar, trying to comfort her a bit by being close to her. There was a moon, but soon big clouds came up and covered it. The night grew very dark. A little red glow came from the fire but that was all. The air grew cold. Rain slashed down and put the fire out and soon Alex and Nelly lay in mud, shivering with cold as well as fear. Both inched their way a little closer to the ashes, hoping their faces and fronts might feel a little warmth even though their backs were freezing. Nelly began to whimper. A voice from inside the hut began to swear. Nelly cried louder, desperate, choking and crying underneath her smelly bandage. Someone crawled out of the doorway, shone a torch onto her face.

'Is that you yowlin' like a cat? If I have to get up again I'll slit your throat. See?'

He turned and shuffled back inside the hut. Alex heard him grunt and snuffle for a while, then snore. Nelly began to sob again. Alex felt her body jerking as she struggled to keep quiet. Somebody swore inside the hut and the man with the torch stumbled back out. He propped his torch on a log and picked up a stick. He slouched over Nelly, who lay still with her eyes squeezed shut. Alex shut his as well.

'I told you, stupid,' the man snarled. 'Now you've

'ad your chips.' He raised his stick and spat.

Alex waited for the sound of the stick hitting his sister. Instead he heard a throaty growl followed by '*Bleedinell!*' He opened his eyes and saw an animal crouched to spring, long dagger teeth bared and glinting in the torchlight. His shadow danced behind him, huge and hunched and threatening. Deep angry snarls rumbled up from the pit of his throat. His eyes, red in the torchlight, glared at the hand that held the stick.

The man dropped it and backed slowly away into the hut, fastening the canvas flap with shaking hands as best he could behind him. 'Bleedinell,' he muttered once more. 'Bloody great creature out there – wolf-hound or summink,' Alex heard him mutter.

'Wot's it doin'?' another voice demanded.

'Gettin' ready to eat them kids by the looks of it.'

'Well, git out there and see to it before it bites their 'eads off.'

'Git out yerself. I ain't goin' nowhere.'

Back outside Nell sat up and pulled her gag down off her mouth. She rubbed her wrists, and said in a small, shaky voice. 'Hello, dog.' The old dog lumbered forward uncertainly. He seemed pleased to see Nelly, his feathered tail swung softly from side to side.

Moonlight showed the sores still raw on his neck but he had lost his look of misery.

'Nell,' Alex whispered. 'Cut me free. Knife in my pocket. Quick.'

Nell sawed away at the bandage between Alex's wrists and when it fell away she gave him the knife. The stuff round her ankles was still tight. Alex cut her feet loose, then his own. They both stood up and both fell down again.

The dog loped over and pushed his big head against Nelly, nosing for chews.

'You've eaten them already,' Nelly told him.

'Run, Nelly. Come on. Before they come out of the shack!'

'I've got pins and needles.'

'Hang onto me and I'll hang onto you.'

They wobbled to their feet and ran. The dog meanwhile had pushed his nose into the pot and was licking up whatever was left in the bottom. He did not follow Nell and Alex.

'How did you get free, Nell?' Alex asked, when they had gone far enough to risk resting a moment.

'My bandages came loose. They didn't tie them properly.'

'Why didn't you tell me?'

'I was too scared to talk.'

'We've got to walk all night now, Nelly. And keep listening out.'

'Will they come after us?'

'They might.'

'I wish the dog would.'

'Maybe he will.'

'I can't see where I'm going.'

'It's lighter than it was. It's almost dawn. If we keep going uphill we'll be heading in the right direction. Gran's place is on the other side of the hill, we're nearly there, Nelly.'

Alex did not say what he was thinking. The worst part of the journey was probably going to be arriving.

Ten

The sun was low down, red and shining in their eyes as they walked down the hill to their grandmother's house. Alex was plodding, worn out, with Nelly on his back. The house looked smaller than last time he'd seen it. The slate roof caught the evening light but the windows looked dark, like watching eyes. Behind the house the sea shone inky black. Alex could hear the waves burst on the rocks and hiss along the stony beach. White foam flew up into the evening sky.

They won't be there, he told himself. *They can't be there.* He said it to Nelly too. '*They're not there, Nelly.*' It sounded cruel but he couldn't let himself or her pretend their parents might be down there, waiting for them, or it would hurt too much to find they weren't. Alex wanted so much to hear his father say: *Well done, Alex. You made it. Now I'm here to do the rest.* To feel his mother's arms round him, her sharp chin pressing on his forehead. He wanted Nelly to want them instead of wanting him. He wanted them to be there.

He eased Nelly down off his back and stood in the road holding her hand. She would have run straight down the hill if Alex hadn't stopped her. Instead, they sat in the shelter of a rock, watching the house for a whole hour. Nelly soon slept. A lonely wind blew off the sea and Alex shivered. By the time a light came on indoors, he was numb. Soon it would be safe to creep down and look through the window. They might be there. They might.

When he was just about ready to make a move, the front door opened and Dandy came out. He looked around and then went back inside. Alex's fear fell away and his eyes filled up with tears of relief. He shook Nelly awake and pointed down the hill.

'Dandy's there,' he said. 'Look, Nelly. Dandy's down there with Gran.'

'Can I go down now?' Nelly asked.

'Not yet. I'll go down first and see if they're alone.'

'That isn't fair.'

'D'you want the police to catch you, Nelly? If they're down there?'

Nelly shook her head and slid her thumb into her mouth. Alex crept down through the heather, and round to the back of the house.

Kate Kentigern and her son Dandy were sitting at the kitchen table. Kate was pouring tea, Dandy was slicing soda bread. Nobody else was there. Alex tapped on the window. When Dandy threw open the kitchen door, the black weight of his fear rolled down off Alex's back and he fell into the warm room and his grandmother's embrace.

The smell of turpentine and wood ash and pipe tobacco reminded Alex of so many childhood visits. All of his grandmother's pictures hung exactly where they always had – the donkey over the mantelpiece, the bluebell woods on the wall opposite, the sunset at sea. The bookcase, the worn-thin rug, the log box, everything was where it belonged. Now he was too. He could smell soup and soda bread and the dusty smell of the dried flowers in the bowl.

'Gran. Nelly's up the hill,' he gasped. Dandy was out and up the hill and back with Nelly in his arms before Alex had finished hugging Kate.

'Where are Ruth and Rob, Alex?' Kate asked, over and over. 'Why aren't they with you?'

Alex shook his head. He couldn't speak. When Nelly came in she slid down out of Dandy's arms and took her grandmother's gnarly hand. 'They got caught, Granny Kate,' she said quietly. 'Some bad men stopped the car and took them away. They hit Dad and they pushed Mum over. Alex brought us here. Some other people helped us. And a dog. But Alex did it mostly.'

Kate put an arm round each of her grandchildren and they clung together as though a gale was blowing cold enough to freeze their hearts. Presently Kate let them go and dried her eyes on her painty overall.

'Dandy's here,' she said. 'Dandy will know what to do.'

Nelly went all round the small house checking every room, looking in each one to make sure, quite sure, that her parents weren't there, somehow, after all. When she knew for certain that they weren't, she curled herself up on her uncle's lap and shut her eyes.

Kate brought soup and bread to them by the fire. Dandy laid Nelly in an armchair with a shawl tucked round her. He wanted to know everything that had happened, how Nell and Alex had coped, where they'd been and who had helped them, everything. But both Nelly and Alex were too tired to talk.

'Let them sleep, Dandy,' Kate said. 'They're worn out. We all are. Talk and make plans in the morning.' She fetched blankets and pillows and tucked Alex and Nelly up together on the sofa. It was big enough that they could both stretch out in comfort.

Alex must already have grown used to listening while he slept because he woke at once when Dandy passed through the front room. After a while he got up and followed him. He wanted to talk without Nelly listening. He guessed Dandy had gone down to the beach to walk and think. He slipped his jacket on, shoved his feet into his muddy shoes and went outside. The moon was up. The little cove looked spectacular. He could see Dandy down on the beach; he went slowly down the path to join him. It would hurt to talk. But it had to be done.

There was a pile of rocks on the way down to the beach and the path wound round them. There was a point in the bend from which the beach could not be seen. Then the path curved round and there it was, like magic. Alex had always loved that moment when he could see the sea again.

Dandy was standing on the beach just looking at the water, when Alex went behind the rocks. When he came out, Dandy was gone. Alex stopped and looked up and down the beach two or three times before he saw him, kneeling in the moonlight. There was something odd about the way he crouched there. He seemed to Alex to be pulling something out of a pocket inside his coat. Or even out of the lining. Alex couldn't see what it was. Moonlight glinted on it and Alex heard the crackle of static. Then Dandy's voice, cool and quiet like it always was.

'The kids have arrived. Walked in of their own accord. I haven't questioned them yet – you can do your own dirty work. Why should they know the foreman's name? They didn't stop long, did they? Their father took the samples and left. You ask them. Pick them up tomorrow.'

Alex slid down to the ground as though someone had punched him. He couldn't think straight, couldn't get his breath. Dandy, his uncle Dandy, Dad's own brother, had betrayed them. How could he do this? Why?

He crept back up that hill bent double and rolled back under the blanket. When Dandy came in, Alex shut his eyes. He felt shocked and stupid but he knew enough to understand that Dandy mustn't know he knew. He heard Dandy stop, felt him looking down. He didn't move a muscle. Nelly sighed in her sleep and turned over. Dandy went upstairs to bed. Alex lay stiff and still on the sofa. He wouldn't tell Nelly about Dandy. But he must tell his grandmother.

Keep me in touch, Dandy had said to his dad. Alex didn't sleep again that night. He didn't dare get up to make a cup of tea, or read a book, or anything, for fear of Dandy creeping down the stairs. All he could think of was the good times, good times with Dandy. Every good time was spoiled now. Worst of all was the knowledge that his dad had trusted Dandy. Who wouldn't trust their own brother? But he lay still and quiet. Because he knew he'd never hide what he felt now. And yet, he managed, in the morning. Said he'd slept well, and smiled. Dandy was on his way out again.

'Going down to the beach to stretch my legs,' he said. This time Alex didn't follow him. Nelly slept on, peaceful and quiet on the sofa.

As soon as Dandy was gone, Alex told his grand-mother. She leaned her weight on the back of a chair, knees sagging, and stared at him. 'You can't be right, Alex. You must be mistaken. Dandy's my son. Rob's brother. Dandy would not betray his brother.'

'He has. And we've got to believe it even if we can't understand it. Because we've got to think what to do.'

'I don't understand. Tell me again, Alex.'

'He said "The kids have turned up. I haven't quest-ioned them. You can do your own dirty work". He said something about the foreman's name – that must be the foreman of the prisoners, where Dad took the samples. He said "Pick them up tomorrow." That's today.'

Kate Kentigern said nothing. She shook her head and stared at Alex. Her face was white with shock; tears welled up in her eyes and trickled down her face. Alex could see she was beginning to believe him. 'He knew about the foreman,' he insisted. 'And the samples. *We* didn't tell him. How did he know it?' He felt cruel, forcing his grandmother to face what Dandy, her own son, had done. But he had to do it.

'Why? Why, Alex?'

'I don't know.'

She sat down, her shoulders shaking with sobs and Alex put his arms round her.

'I won't believe he did this of his own free will, Alex. Not Dandy. It's not possible and I won't believe it.'

'Whatever made him do it, Gran, we have to think about what to do next. We have to decide now. Don't we?'

Kate Kentigern nodded and blew her nose. Neither of them had noticed Nelly waking up. She sat quite still with her face going first white, then red.

'He said he would take care of us,' she said quietly. 'But he was telling lies. I hope he dies, Alex.'

'That's not very nice, Nell,' Dandy said from the doorway. 'Is it?'

Eleven

Alex looked at his uncle's face and saw it was too late to lie his way out of trouble. Dandy ignored him and spoke to Kate. 'The police will be here shortly,' he said. 'Alex and Nelly will be taken care of. Nobody's going to harm them. They promised me that much.'

Kate Kentigern was silent for a long time, so long that Alex thought she wasn't going to say anything. When at last she spoke, she looked Dandy in the eye. 'In return for what, Dandy? What did you promise them? And why? You've done a wicked thing, Dandy. But you have goodness in you still, and strength. Use them both now. Let the children go.'

'I can't.' Dandy shook his head miserably.

'I know as much as they do, Dandy. Whatever it is the police want to know, you and I can tell them. Let the children go.'

Dandy looked at his mother, then looked away. His face was full of pain.

'They took Rachel,' he said. 'They've got her still. She's only safe while I do what they say. I had no choice.'

'There is always a choice, Dandy,' Kate told him.

There was no time for her to say more. A car came grinding down the hill road and braked noisily. Two men got out and barged in at the door. Kate Kentigern held out her hand with icy formality and stared imperiously at the policemen, who ignored her. Dandy stood by, his face red with shame, as the police grabbed Alex and Nelly and hauled them out to the car. Nelly fought back, her small face blotched with tears. 'Don't fight, Nelly,' Dandy begged. 'Do what they say. They won't hurt you, I promise.'

'Liar!' Nelly shouted.

Kate grabbed her old jacket and followed her grandchildren. All three prisoners were bundled into the back of the car. One policeman sat in the front seat and muttered into his radio. He seemed to be discussing which roads to take with somebody. The other went back to the house to speak to Dandy. He returned after a few minutes and they drove off, leaving the door to Kate Kentigern's house swinging open in the rising wind off the sea, and Dandy standing alone, staring after them.

Rocking and bouncing in the back of the car between his sister and his grandmother, Alex tried not to think about what was coming next. Nelly was hunched down in her seat and shaking. Alex found her hand and gripped it tightly. Surely, Alex thought, they won't hurt Nelly. Surely, they won't hurt Gran. But he knew already that he and Nelly and their grandmother were not, in these men's eyes, a boy, a girl and an old woman, frightened, maybe frail. They were not part of a family, with loving ties, quarrels and hopes and fears. They were not part of anything these men recognised. They were not people, they were enemies. And once that happens, anything can follow.

One of the men lit up. Used smoke filled the car and Alex felt his stomach heave as they swung round each bend.

'Would you mind opening a window?' Kate Kentigern asked. 'If you must smoke.'

'Well pardon me for breathing,' the driver mocked.

'I don't know where you're taking us. Or why,' Kate Kentigern replied. 'But I see no reason why we should breathe your foul smog in the meantime.'

The man beside the driver looked round. 'Worried

about your health are you? Well I'll tell you this just once. If you *are*, you'll do what you're told. Shut it.'

'Never mind, Granny,' Nelly whispered. 'Don't take any notice. It's just a bit smelly, that's all.'

'And keep those brats shtum too,' the man grunted. 'Unless you want 'em to feel the back of my hand.'

After that they drove in silence, apart from the odd crackle of the car radio checking on their whereabouts. Presently the car swung off down a narrow road that led into a small plantation. Pine trees grew close on either side. The wind was strengthening, blowing wild off the Atlantic, combing the heather on the hills and screaming through the trees, making them lean, rise up, and lean again as each blast hit them. The sky was huge, with pools of green between the ragged clouds. A spatter of hailstones hit the windscreen, the crack of it making Alex jump. The driver, too, seemed jumpy.

'Damn rain. Bloody road. Out in the godforsaken sticks,' he cursed. 'Who the hell lives out here anyway?' He put his foot down, eager to get out from under the trees and head back towards main roads and towns.

Even above the engine and the wind they all heard it – a creak that grew into a rending, tearing, splintering crash at the same time as the rough red trunk of a pine tree sliced down through birch and bracken, hit the road ahead and bounced. The driver swore again and braked. Alex shot forward, hitting his head on the back of the seat in front. He felt a salty trickle of blood start down his lip. Nelly was doubled up beside him, forehead to knees, unhurt, her grandmother's arms round her.

The two men in front got out and kicked the big tree ineffectually. The driver fetched a crowbar out of the boot to use as a lever. His mate stood by and fiddled with a gun he'd taken from under his seat. Alex tried to calculate what chance they had of making it, if they got out and ran. No chance. Even on his own he wouldn't make more than a few yards.

The back door opened and a hand reached in.

'Get out and make yourself useful. We've got to shift this tree trunk.' Alex got out. On either side of the road the trees stretched back, row on tidy row, like pillars in a dark cathedral. A little undergrowth straggled up towards the light but there was not much cover. Up in the roof of the wood, wind stormed and branches rocked. Glancing up the long rows on either side, Alex noticed a rope trailing from the top of the tree that blocked the road. The driver hadn't seen it yet. Alex forced himself to look away. That's when he saw two feet wearing good boots, and the tip of an arrow, protruding from a bramble bush. Madoc's boots. Madoc's arrow. Above the bush, high in a pine tree, Anna sat looking down at him, her crossbow on her lap. He looked away. Looked back at Nelly and his grandmother still huddled in the back of the police car.

Should he run? Make a diversion? But if he did, he would be shot before he got off the road. What then? He hesitated for a second, not allowing himself to look either at Madoc, or at Anna, or at the rope on the tree. In that second Anna raised her bow and the man with the gun folded over and slid onto the ground, his back against the shiny car door and a dozen or more people, with Madoc at the front, charged yelling out of the wood.

Kate Kentigern was helped out of the car, shaking. 'It's all right, Granny,' Nelly told her. 'They're friends.' Anna scrambled down out of the tree. Somebody got the crowbar off the remaining policeman, tied him up and put him in the back of his car. How sudden it can be, that change from guard to prisoner. Everything that might be useful was taken from the car – maps, radios, the gun, even a bag of peppermints and a flask of tea.

The man Anna had shot was dead. They lifted him into the car too. Alex watched. He had seen the young woman die in a hospital bed, killed by disease. Now he had seen a man shot dead. He would have killed me, Alex thought. And Gran. And Nelly, if somebody told him to. Somehow, it didn't make much difference. The man had been alive. Now he was dead. Even the death of a bad man, Alex thought, leaves a big gap. But the body looked heavy and dead; nothing more. Will was told to drive the car away and leave it where it would be found. 'Which is more than they would do for us,' he grumbled.

'Aren't we more than them, Will?' Madoc asked.

Will shrugged, climbed in and drove away.

'How did you know where we were?' Alex asked.

'Heard it on the radio,' Madoc answered. 'We listen in. Two young ones and an old lady, picked up in Gartbeg. It had to be you.'

'What will happen to my son Dandy?' Kate Kentigern asked. 'And Rachel, poor Rachel, what will they do to her?'

Madoc shook his head.

'He's not wicked, my Dandy's not,' Kate said quietly. 'Just a muddler.'

'Of course he's not,' Madoc agreed. 'Most of us bend when they start to twist us.'

Kate sat down slowly by the road, wet grass and mud dabbling her heavy skirt.

'How could I not have realised about Rachel?' she wept. 'How could I have thought him capable of that? How will he bear to think I ever thought it?'

Madoc bent over her. 'Folk may help him,' he told her. 'Him and his wife. Never give up.'

'Thank you,' Kate said, when she could speak. 'For helping my grandchildren before, and for helping us now.' One of her long white plaits had come loose and was dangling down her back. Her hands shook, and her paint-smeared apron flapped in the cold wind. 'I'm not sure what we're going to do now,' she said.

Alex, watching her, saw that she was old and frightened.

Twelve

They walked for half the day, over heather and under rowan trees, beside a slate-dark loch, along the rocky edge of a peat-brown burn. At first wet bracken soaked them but they climbed until they were above it, slowly, steadily. Nelly grumbled. Kate did not. Late in the afternoon they sat down to rest below a high ridge. Pine trees straggled round its feet. Above them, purple heather, and then grey scree ran up between great folded walls of crumpled granite. Water came down cold and clear and Nelly kicked her shoes off to bathe her hot feet.

'Can we stay here?' she asked. 'For a bit?'

'We'll stay here till it's dark,' Brigid told her.

'Then what?'

'Where we go next is a secret. No one must see.'

Alex helped Anna brew tea – bitter and black as usual – and pass it round with hunks of bread Brigid pulled out of a sack. Kate Kentigern leaned back against a rock and lit her pipe.

'I'd like to paint that,' she said, looking up at the ridge. Her head tipped forward, her eyes closed, and she snored.

Once it was dusk, Madoc woke everyone who had managed to sleep, called in the guards he'd posted, and got everyone together. 'Listen,' he said. 'We're going home. You know what that means. It means quiet. It means watch where you tread. It means leave no mark behind you in the heather. When we get the signal, Brigid answers. The rest of us are silent. Ready?'

They all moved off with Brigid in front, Kate, Alex and Nelly and Anna somewhere in the middle of the line and Madoc at the back. They climbed, slowly, silently, one foot in front of the other, while the small moon climbed the sky beside them. When Nelly could climb no more she was passed from back to back. Alex and Anna walked with Kate Kentigern between them. By and by she put one arm around each of their necks and they half-carried, half-towed her up the mountain side. Startled sheep bounced away down the slope. When the cloud cleared and the moon gave a bit of light, Alex saw that the trees were way below them. A narrow path wound between rock and heather up over the shoulder of the mountain. A mountain hare, brown now in her summer coat, shot off, lifted in long bounds. Alex could hear water falling. The ground above seemed to flatten into a cup, like the palm of a hand, with a cliff of rock at the back of it and scree at the front. Madoc walked them up into the palm.

They stopped in the green hollow and Alex heard somebody whistle. Brigid answered, and they went on. This happened twice more, and they seemed about to leave the cup of green behind. Ahead the rock rose sheer. Alex could see no path, nor any place a path could lead to, beyond the mass of grey rock that tumbled out from the base of the cliff. A grove of stunted rowan trees clung to the rocks, seeming to grow straight out of them, with low crowberry bushes hiding their roots.

Madoc took them in under the trees. Red berries hung down all around and Nelly, riding high on Anna's back, reached up her hand and picked some. Behind her, Kate Kentigern smiled. She knew why Nelly wanted rowan berries. Rowan berries keep off witches. Almost Kate thought she'd pick some too, the place they grew in was so strange. She looked up at the glossy bunched berries and the slim green leaves. When she looked back, Madoc had disappeared. Anna took her arm and pulled her forward.

Kate found herself walking into the mountain, between two overhanging rocks. She smelled wood smoke and sweat and wet clothes and knew that she was close to many people. 'Granny,' Nelly whispered. 'Granny, what's happening?' Kate reached up and patted Nelly's cheek, but did not speak. Together they pushed past a smelly curtain of deer hides, and then another. Past the second curtain, the glow from a fire pit and the light of a few candles showed a ring of people sitting in a high, smoke-blackened cave.

High on the cave wall rusted metal brackets held a worn flagpole. An ancient, tattered banner swung gently in the small heat rising from the crowd below. 'Jacobites hung that there, after Culloden,' Anna whispered to Alex.

One and another of the cave folk looked up and greeted Madoc's crowd. Room was made for them by the fire pit, and a place for Kate on a rough wooden bench. 'You're safe here,' Brigid said. 'You're with the runners. You can rest now.'

By the time Madoc's crowd were all awake the guards outside the cave had come and gone several times. It was midmorning, and a wet one. Whenever someone came past the deer-hide curtain they would pause to shake themselves before stamping over to the little peat fire. Nobody ever dried out, and the cave smelled of peat smoke and wet wool and worse.

Anna woke and crawled out from under her blanket. Someone was making tea and she brought some to Alex.

'Is this your home?' he asked. 'When you're not in the woods?'

'Sort of. Not all the time. We stay a while, when we need to keep out of sight mostly, and then we leave. But I've not been back to my real home in a long while. My real home is Galashiels, a long way south from here.'

'Why did you leave?'

'Madoc got caught selling petrol on the black market.'

'I thought everybody did that.'

'Not everyone gets caught though, do they? And it depends who you are. And who you know. We had to leave. Brigid knows everybody. She knew how to find the runners. We've been with them ever since.'

'The dancing pin man sign – is that the runners' sign?'

'It's a freedom sign. The runners are for freedom. If you're for freedom, you're for the dancing man. He's everywhere. So are the runners. There's even some down south in England now, they say. And Wales and Ireland too.'

Alex, Nelly, Kate Kentigern and Madoc's crowd stayed in the cave ten days, going out only at dusk and dawn. People brought in meat – sheep once, a deer, sometimes a hare. Alex took his turn alongside Madoc on guard duty to learn how it should be done. During that time folk came and went, as Anna said they would. At dawn on their eleventh day, guards whistled to let those inside know a friend was coming, and a young woman swung in under the curtain. She was tired and wet through but elated. She brought news of big troubles down in Glasgow. People had rioted, groups were leaving the city in large numbers, some going south into the Moorfoot Hills, some coming north. New groups of runners were growing everywhere. The best news of all was that a squad of men sent out from Paisley to catch stragglers had run off with them instead to start a camp of their own.

'If the soldiers are deserting, we're in business,' Madoc said.

The questions Madoc had sent out, asking for news of Ruth and Rob, had been answered. It seemed that they were working on the self-same stretch of road from which they'd taken samples.

'That must be done from spite,' Brigid reckoned. 'They're too old to be working on the roads.'

'The foreman will help them,' Alex said.

'The foreman won't be there,' Madoc replied. 'He's gone. They caught him letting prisoners escape.'

Alex remembered his big, open laugh. Most likely, Alex thought, he wouldn't laugh much any more.

Madoc began at once to make plans for their rescue. He said he would take Anna, with her crossbow, plus a couple of newcomers. And Alex. Nelly raged at being made to stay behind.

'It isn't fair you're going to see them first. Let me come too. I won't get in the way, I promise!'

Alex and the rest departed, leaving Nelly sobbing. Kate held her tightly in her arms and rocked her. Later, when Nelly slept, Kate lit her pipe and smoked a while, then begged an old paper bag from Brigid which she smoothed out and began to draw on, using a pencil stub she had in her pocket.

It was a three day trek to get back in striking distance

of the motorway, travelling carefully. They timed it to arrive an hour or two before the midnight shift–change. Alex hid in a ditch beside Anna and watched, waiting for Madoc to give the signal. He saw his mother and father at once, bent over, working slowly, two figures dressed in prison rags, splashed head to foot in red mud, a glint of metal showing at their wrists. Beside them worked the twins Alex had seen before. Rob shovelled gravel into a cement mixer. Ruth was loading a wheelbarrow. Every time she filled it, it was wheeled away and another was brought up, leaving her no time to straighten up between barrows.

Seeing them there, exhausted, dirty, diminished by their prison rags, Alex felt anger swamp his fear. How dare anybody do this to them? Then he remembered it was Dandy who had done it, out of fear for Rachel. Who pulled Dandy's strings then? Who sat up at the top of the whole dirty pile? Alex pushed such complexities away. What mattered now was to get them off the roads, away from the sickness, out with the runners. He caught himself, for a brief second, thinking of his parents as people he was going to risk his life to help. Before, he'd been their child, relied on *them* to keep *him* safe. Now, he must try to keep them safe.

Alex carried no weapon other than a sheath knife.

He did not know how to shoot a crossbow or fire a gun. He was pretty sure he couldn't stick a knife into anybody, but Madoc had told him that he'd be surprised what he could do, when push came to shove. He realised now that Madoc was right. Anna had been able to shoot the policeman with her crossbow. Quite likely, Alex thought, he'd do the same now, if he could.

Madoc gave the signal and Anna shot the lights out on the tower. Alex, Madoc and the two men threw themselves onto the road. Madoc knocked the new foreman off his feet and pinned him to the ground. Prisoners dived everywhere, flickering like cartoon characters in the lights of passing cars. Ruth and Rob saw Alex simultaneously. Too amazed to run, they flung their arms round him, clinging, hugging, gasping. Alex tugged himself free and then all three of them were diving through the mud and rubble, skidding and rolling down the bank, pelting across the field.

They stopped for a second in the shelter of a hedge and looked back. Alex saw Anna, still up on the road, pushing the twins in front of her, yelling to the rest to run. Somewhere a siren screeched. Madoc thumped down next to Alex in the dark. 'Right, lad,' he growled. 'We're off. Don't stop for anybody now.'

Long after he thought his lungs would burst, Alex

ran. Ruth and Rob ran with him. They ran until Madoc told them they could stop. Then they dropped straight down onto the wet ground, gasping, arms tight round one another. It was only when they stood up and let go that Alex noticed Anna wasn't there. Madoc would not come back without her. 'You go on,' he told his two men. 'Alex – tell Brigid that I'll find Anna.'

Alex's joy at being with his parents was cut through with fear for Anna. But he was proud to tell, talking as they walked, how he'd managed to bring Nelly safe to their grandmother in Gartbeg. What he had to tell them about Dandy made them all ashamed. Ashamed for Dandy, for what he had been forced to do once Rachel was taken. Guilty, as though the guilt was theirs. Fearful. What would he have done, Rob asked himself, if Ruth had been the hostage? What would happen now, to Dandy, when his bosses found out he had failed?

When, finally, three days later they passed the guards and pushed in under the deer hide curtains, Ruth and Rob stood still, looking across the dark and smoky space to where Nelly lay sleeping on a pile of blankets. Kate Kentigern looked up from her place by the fire. Her lined face opened out in happiness. She stood, embraced her son, kissed Ruth, hugged Alex. Rob, hugging her, saw how her face was sharper, thinner, older than it had been. But she smiled, and pointed to where Nelly lay, wrapped in an old sheepskin, her thumb in her mouth, fast asleep by the fire.

Ruth sat down quietly beside her. Presently a log in the fire cracked, sending sparks swarming up towards the rock roof of the cave. Nelly woke, glanced at the fire, looked up, and saw her mother looking down at her. She didn't cry, or laugh, or say a word. She wriggled over to Ruth's arms and clung for a long time with her face pressed against Ruth's neck, her forehead butting under Ruth's chin, her arms tight round Ruth's neck.

Every now and then, Ruth would reach out one hand and pull Alex close so she could sit with an arm round each of them. Rob sat at her back, one hand over her shoulder, twisting a strand of Nelly's soft hair in his fingers, glancing across her small head now and then to grin at Alex with delighted pride. Feeling his mother's arm across his shoulders, his father's pride, and Nelly, safe at last, Alex felt something like a mountain roll off his tired back.

Later, Kate joined them. Alex and Nelly slept, while Rob, Ruth and Kate Kentigern talked out their pity and their shock. *Poor Dandy. Oh, poor Rachel. What's happening to her, do you think? How could he do it? How could he not? How will it be, when we see him again?* In the end they agreed that he was family. That none of them knew what they would have done, if they'd been him. That they must forgive him. That they never could.

'Not in the real sense,' Ruth said, sadly. 'If not blaming, if trying to understand, means forgiving, I can do that. But if it means loving him again, trusting him again, I can't.'

'I can,' Kate Kentigern said. 'And I will.'

Brigid meanwhile was still red-eyed from crying over Anna. She was still missing and nobody had any news of where she might be. She had brought the twins down to the hedge and then run back for someone else. She had not come back across the field to run with the rest of them. That was all anybody knew.

Madoc came in a few days after Alex and his parents, rested a day, then took Will and went back to search again. He came back a fortnight later with a rumour that she had been sent south to a big new prison. He rested, heard what news there was, then left again.

It was a hard time, and worst of all for Brigid, with Anna and Madoc gone and no word of what might be happening to them. Anna was a prisoner; that much was certain. A bent, spent figure working on a road somewhere.

'She'll know we're looking for her,' Brigid said. 'She knows we won't give up. And we won't be the only ones. We've got folk everywhere now, doing what they can. There'll be runners somewhere about, wherever she's been put, doing what they can for prisoners in their region. Anna knows that. She won't give up hope.'

Alex suffered privately. Blamed himself for running with his parents instead of waiting for her. Begged Madoc when he next returned to let him search as well.

'Thank you for offering, lad,' Madoc told him. 'But you don't know enough yet. You'd be no help.' Alex blushed, and waited. He was the first beside the fire when any news came in, the first to hear what any cold, wet traveller had to tell.

Kate Kentigern suffered as well, but she did not complain of anything, except when she ran out of paper or tobacco. She was afraid for Dandy and his Rachel. She seemed to shrink inside her bundle of clothes until, tall as she was, she weighed little more than Nelly. She longed to go home, but Brigid wouldn't hear of it.

'Not safe,' she said. 'They'll be watching the place. We'll take you to a safe place soon – a house with a bit o'comfort. But not your own house. And not yet.'

Most of the prisoners who had got away with Ruth and Rob were brought up to the cave and then passed on from one camp to another, spreading out the burden of the sickness everybody knew must come. Only the twins stayed on in the cave. They were too ill to move. They did not speak, excepting to each other, and that in a peculiar chirping code nobody else could follow.

'Who knows where they've been or what they've seen,' Brigid would sigh, wiping their dirty faces, spooning soup into their bowls. 'Better for us that they can't say, maybe.'

Winter began, with snow on the heather and wind that cut like knives. Down in the valley the loch froze and thick frost furred the rowan trees. Brigid said it was time to move south. Anna would know where they were, and come to them, she said. Two nights before they were to leave, Maggie tramped in with Dayo on her back. People had come out from Stepgavie, she said, moved in and driven her away. Others had guided her on to Madoc's people. To Nelly's great delight, Ludo came with them. He bore the scars of his dogfight, and limped a bit, but otherwise he seemed unscathed.

135

'Where have you been, Deputy Dawg? How did you find Maggie and Dayo?' Nelly demanded, arms tight round his neck. But Ludo wasn't telling.

'He's a runners' dog now,' Maggie laughed. 'He knows who his friends are and what's good for him. He found me, and he stayed with me.'

That night, heavy snow fell, making the descent from the cave too difficult to tackle.

'Fine,' said Madoc, who now had runners down south looking for Anna. 'No one will bother hunting rebels while the snow lasts. We're safe here while the snow lies and all the roads are blocked.'

Alex shot his first buck with Madoc's bow and arrows. They built the fire up high, fearing no passing eyes, and ate it roasted, with singing and music.

The twins died during the snow time. Everyone knew it was coming. They lay together by the fire, taking sips of tea from Brigid or Kate Kentigern. They'd stopped trying to eat some days before, and soon they could not even keep tea down. Brigid and Kate washed them in water heated on the fire, sat with them, held them, sang to them. They lay still, holding one another's hands, with their eyes shut. Only occasionally did one or other of them stare up at whichever face was bending over theirs. Ruth had no medicine with which to ease their deaths. The twins died in the morning, before first light, and were buried the same day – not underneath the earth. The earth was frozen hard under nearly a metre of snow. Instead, the runners laid the two small bodies down together, wrapped a rug around them, put a sprig of heather in their hands, and built a cairn of stones above their bodies. Brigid wept, fearing that Anna might be making the selfsame journey herself, and alone maybe, without people round her to wish her goodbye. Alex cried too, alone in the darkness outside the cave where nobody could see.

After the burial, Kate and Brigid sang. Two lads had snare drums, someone else a fiddle. Sparks rose with the music and the rock overhead seemed to shift and breathe in the flame light. Out above the mountain, the sky made a roof of black over the white.

Gradually the evening ended. Nelly stuffed a last piece of venison into her mouth and wiped her hand down the front of her coat. Brigid fetched snow from outside ready to melt for water in the morning. Somebody had a bag of chestnuts. Madoc pierced them on the point of his knife and dropped them into the edge of the fire to cook among the ashes. One or two popped. A dog yipped in its sleep. The people all were quiet.

Out in the darkness, someone whistled. Anna's two terriers rose and trotted out, tails erect and small ears cocked. The figures round the fire looked up. For a moment, the cave waited. A small wind sighed through the deer hide curtains, shifting them stiffly with a cold breath. Other than that nothing stirred. There was no sound except the soft rustle of the fire.

A bent, familiar figure ducked under the curtain and trudged into the fire glow, accompanied by a small snow flurry. She reached the fire, slid slowly down onto her knees and held her hands out to the warmth. Faces turned towards her, warm red in the firelight.

'It's beginning,' Anna said. 'The towns are nearly empty. Soldiers are coming over too. They say by spring the whole of Scotland will be for the dancing man.'

Alex leaned towards her. He put his hand up to her dirty, wind-chapped cheek. He forgot about fighting and freedom. He forgot about Madoc and Brigid. He forgot about his parents, watching from the shadows. He forgot everything for a while, except only that Anna was safe.

There was a dragon in the sky the night before the stranger came. It flamed across the red west from the cliffs to the black road of the sea. Its jaws were open, showing its curved teeth tinged with yellow. The single eye it turned towards me glowed like an ember in the darkness of its face. I watched it while the sun went down and its body bleached from fire to gold to crumpled leather. I watched it till the sun was gone. It must have slid down to the land of ice then, because I could see no more of it. But all the time I saw it in the sky, I know it saw me too. Its red eye watched my grey eye. It did not speak to me. But I feared it.

In the morning when I woke, I felt a new thing round my neck. Someone had hung a little silver hammer there, to bring me luck and keep me safe.

Amma, my grandmother, got up while it was dark, but I could always find her. I would run down to the beach and see the dark shape of her, with her thick cloak moving in the breeze, her back to the big rock and her face to the ocean. She liked to stand there and think about my grandfather. That rock is where she stood to watch him leave, the last time that he sailed away.

Perhaps he feasts with Ran now. Perhaps my father and my brothers feast there with him. Or, if they all died fighting, they'll be in Odin's great hall. I hope they didn't die some other way and go down to the land of Hel. I doubt if there's much feasting at her table.

'Amma!' I shouted. 'Amma! Look what Thor has brought me in the night!'

I knew, and Amma knew I knew, that it was she who put the hammer there. But with Amma I spoke as I felt. And I felt sure that Thor had made her do it, because he cared for me. I was a child then, though I was sixteen.

My name is Ran. Amma named me Ran because I love the sea – and maybe for my stormy temper. Ran is the goddess of the sea; she pulls the drowning sailors down to her great hall at the bottom of the ocean. Sometimes I hate my name because it's hers, but Amma says I mustn't.

'The gods do what they must do, Ran,' she used to say, 'the same as us.'

'Why be a god then, Amma?' I would ask.

'They are who they must be. Now stand here and pay attention. The border of your weaving's a disgrace.'

We were not rich, my people, but we were not poor. We had our fields, and the fishing from the sea. We kept cattle, half a dozen, sheep and three pigs, goats, and a flock of chickens. And Bor, my father's horse, though he was already old then. Our farm was called Smolsund. We had no slaves, and only one servant to help us, an old man we called Od.